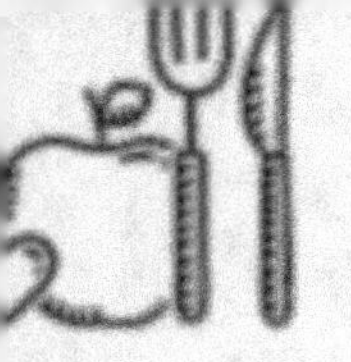

LEAN AFTER 50

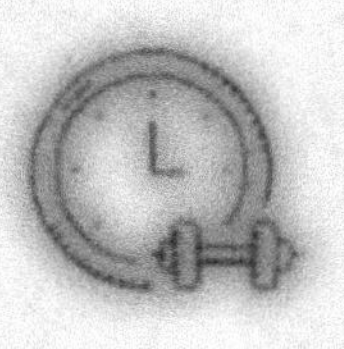
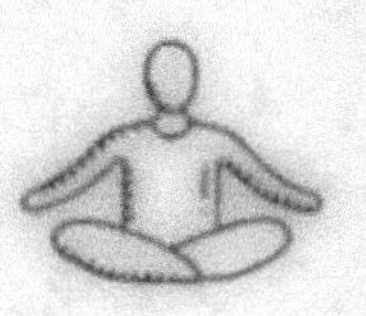
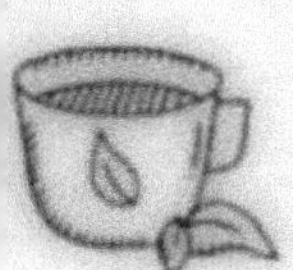

A COMPREHENSIVE GUIDE TO FITNESS, NUTRITION, AND LONGEVITY

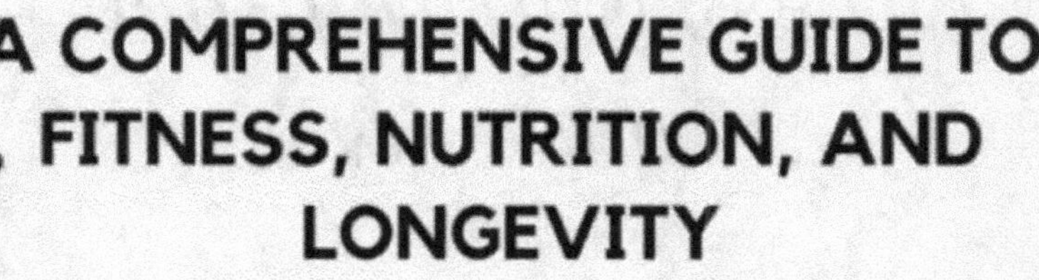
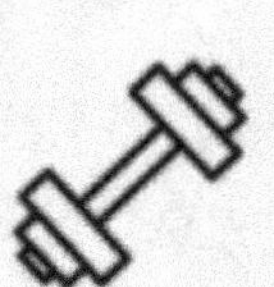

Unlock the secrets to vitality and longevity after 50 – it's time to thrive in your best years

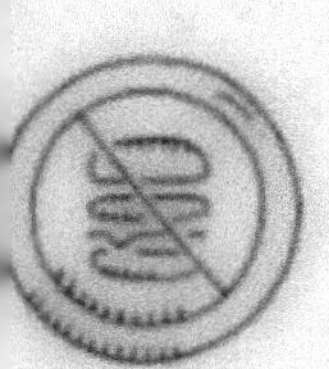
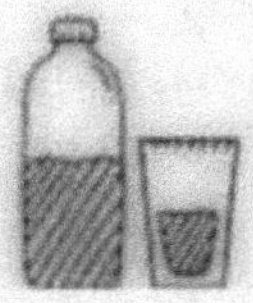
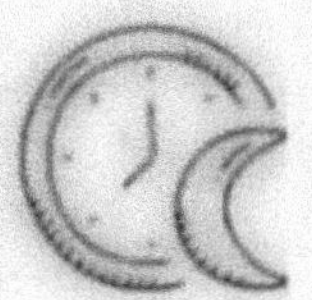

NATALIE BECK

LEAN AFTER 50

A Comprehensive Guide to Fitness, Nutrition, and Longevity

Natalie Beck

Table of Content

Introduction

Imagine waking up every day feeling tired before you even get out of bed. For many over the age of 50, this is a harsh reality. The morning routine is a struggle, battling aches and pains, and the energy that once fueled your days feels like a distant memory. As the hours pass, the grind of daily life takes its toll—long hours sitting at a desk, consuming processed foods, and the mounting stress of responsibilities. By evening, your body screams for rest. Many find themselves collapsing on the couch, too fatigued to engage in physical activities.

But it's not just about physical exhaustion. Over time, this lifestyle leads to the insidious creeping in of weight gain, loss of muscle mass, and a feeling of helplessness. These aren't just numbers on a scale; they're markers of a health crisis. The risk of chronic diseases such as diabetes, heart disease, and osteoporosis skyrockets. Health becomes a game of maintenance rather than vitality. And with each passing year, the mountain to climb seems steeper, casting a shadow over the golden years of life.

This scenario isn't just hypothetical. Consider the millions who grapple with these challenges daily. According to the CDC, nearly 40% of adults aged 50 and older are obese, a condition linked to a myriad of health complications. This isn't just about aesthetics—it's about quality of life. The potential for vibrant, active living is buried under layers of unhealthy habits and misinformation.

But let's delve deeper into the pain points. The first major barrier is **misinformation**. The internet is a minefield of quick fixes and fad diets that promise miraculous transformation. They often overlook the unique needs of those over 50, creating frustration and false hope. Then there's **motivation**. How do you find the drive to change when the past attempts have only led to short-lived success? It's easy to feel stuck, as though the effort isn't worth the seemingly marginal gains.

Moreover, there's the issue of **time**. With careers, family obligations, and everyday demands, finding time to focus on health can feel impossible. The gym becomes a distant dream, and meal planning feels like a Herculean task. And let's not forget the **mental barrier**. Exercise and nutrition can feel overwhelming and complex, especially when the body doesn't respond as it did in younger years.

Here's where this book steps in. *Lean After 50: A Comprehensive Guide to Fitness, Nutrition, and Longevity* is not about unrealistic promises. It's about practical, sustainable strategies rooted in science. My goal is to demystify the process of getting fit and staying healthy after 50. We'll explore **the basics of exercise, tailored nutrition plans,** and **mindset shifts** that drive long-term change. You don't need to overhaul your life in a day. Small, consistent steps can lead to profound changes.

In these pages, we'll cover several critical components. First, **you'll learn the essential exercises tailored for your body's needs.** No more confusing gym jargon—just straightforward guidance on movements that build strength and flexibility. Next, we'll examine **nutrition**—not just what to eat, but when to eat and why it matters. You'll understand how macronutrients and hydration play a pivotal role in your health. We'll also address **supplements** and how they can support your journey.

A unique aspect of this book is its focus on **mental resilience and adaptability**. Change begins in the mind, and we'll explore strategies to build and maintain motivation. We'll discuss real-life examples and evidence-based practices that have helped others achieve remarkable transformation.

So, buckle up and commit to this journey. It won't be a quick fix, but it will be a rewarding and transformative one. Whether you've been active all your life or are just starting, there's something here for you. Together, we can rewrite your health story, one chapter at a time.

CHAPTER 1

Fifty & Fit - Basics to the Art of Staying Lean

"Age is no barrier. It's a limitation you put on your mind."

Jackie Joyner-Kersee

Most people think staying fit and healthy after 50 is a losing battle. Perhaps the notion that it's too late to start or that it's inevitable to experience physical decline at this age is the reason behind this belief. I get it—I really do.

You've spent decades nurturing careers, raising families, and finally, you're supposed to kick back. But what if I told you that this is the perfect time to focus on *you*? You're in the driver's seat, and your experience gives you an edge.

Let me paint a picture. Imagine Sandra, a 56-year-old accountant who once believed that her best days were behind her. Like many, Sandra struggled with weight gain, joint pain, and low energy. She felt trapped, thinking it was too late to make a change. Then she tried something radical—a blend of targeted exercise and mindful eating. Within a year, Sandra lost 30 pounds, gained muscle, and became my client, the go-to example of health in our community. How did she do it?

Fitness and Nutrition. Think about them as two sides of a coin. One without the other isn't nearly as powerful. When Sandra incorporated strength training, her muscle mass increased, leading to a higher metabolism even when she wasn't working out.

Did you know that after 50, muscle mass declines by 1-2% per year if unaddressed? Nutrition completes the other half of this puzzle. It's often said that abs are made in the kitchen, and this holds for all age groups. But after 50, our bodies require fewer calories, so choosing nutrient-dense foods that provide energy and support overall health is crucial.

There are two roads from here on. One leads to a downward spiral - increased fat mass leading to more weight gain, higher risk of chronic diseases like diabetes and heart disease, and a reduced quality of life. The other road is the one Sandra took—the uphill path. The first few steps are the hardest—making lifestyle changes can be hard. But once you're there, you're less likely to give up as the results start manifesting. You'll sleep better, experience less joint pain, and feel confident in your body.

A balanced diet and regular exercise aren't fads; they're lifestyle changes that come with a range of benefits. From improved mental health—thanks to endorphins released during exercise—to better sleep patterns, the perks are endless. Picture your body as a high-performance machine. The better you maintain it, the better it performs.

One last thing. You might think—"This sounds like so much work." But think of it as an investment, one that yields returns in the form of energy, happiness, and longevity. Look at real data - the *Harvard Alumni Study* found that those who were physically active by the age of 50 were significantly healthier in their later years.

You don't need to overhaul your life overnight. Small, consistent changes make the difference. Whether it's a 30-minute walk or adding more greens to your plate, every step counts. It might seem daunting at first, but trust me; you'll look back and wonder why you didn't start sooner.

In this first chapter, we'll go over the misconceptions and the basics—the why, the how, and the benefits. Let's dive in!

Addressing Common Misconceptions and Challenges

Growing older is like unfolding a new chapter in the book of life—full of surprises, experiences, and, yes, misconceptions. Let's tackle a few myths that frequently trip people up and stand in the way of their fitness goals.

It's Never Too Late to Start

Consider Ernestine Shepherd as an example. She started bodybuilding at age 56 and went on to become the world's oldest competitive female bodybuilder at the age of 80. Sounds like a Hollywood script, doesn't it? But it's real.

You might think, "I've never been a gym person," or "This is just not me." Yet, the evidence is clear - **starting exercise at any age is beneficial**. Studies by the National Institutes of Health show that even those who begin exercising later in life can significantly improve cardiovascular health, muscle strength, and mental well-being.

When you start, think of it like planting a tree. The best time to plant one was years ago, but the second best time is now. You're not limited by age, but by the decisions you make today.

Safety in Activity

Another common fear - "Exercise is risky for older people." The truth? **Exercise is risky if you don't do it right.** But so is sitting down all day. The American College of Sports Medicine has shown that supervised, low-impact activities like walking, swimming, or yoga can significantly reduce the risk of heart disease and improve joint health.

The doctor is the best person to provide clearance for any major lifestyle change. Ask them how you can safely start incorporating exercise into your routine. Certain conditions, such as arthritis or diabetes, might require specific modifications to your workout plan. But don't worry—there's always a safe and effective way.

More Isn't Always Better

We've all heard of the phrase "no pain, no gain." But that doesn't apply here. In fact, **excessive exercise can be**

harmful for older adults. Our bodies have different needs as we age, and recovery time is longer. Pushing too hard can lead to injuries and setbacks. Finding a balance between pushing yourself and listening to your body is key.

Instead of going all-in, start with manageable goals and gradually increase intensity. Don't be afraid to take rest days and incorporate activities like stretching or yoga on those days. Remember, the goal is longevity, not a short-term fix.

Weight Gain Isn't Inevitable

Let's debunk another myth. Many people throw up their hands and say, "Weight gain is just part of aging." Not quite. Sure, metabolism slows down as you age. But this doesn't mean you have to pile on the pounds.

Yes. The circumstances are mostly true—after 50, *metabolism does slow down*, and our bodies require fewer calories. But this doesn't mean that we can't maintain a healthy weight and body composition. With proper exercise and nutrition, weight gain can be prevented or even reversed.

To sum it up, addressing these misconceptions head-on equips you with the knowledge **to make smarter, healthier choices**. The journey to staying lean isn't about the past limitations you think you have. It's about the potential that's still in you, just waiting to be unlocked.

Understanding the Real Challenges

Let's say you're sitting on a park bench, watching kids dash around with boundless energy, and you can't help but smile. But then you stand up, and an ache in your knee jolts through your body—a stark reminder that getting older isn't for the faint of heart.

While the enthusiasm of undertaking a healthier lifestyle may be present, a certain inherent apprehension might linger. Understanding the real challenges that come with aging can help you develop a targeted plan to overcome them.

Reduced Mobility

Let's consider reduced mobility first. It's a common roadblock, especially with conditions like arthritis or osteoporosis. As we age, our bones and joints naturally get weaker, making physical activity difficult. This is partly due to the synovial fluid in our joints—responsible for lubricating and cushioning them—decreasing with age. This results is more friction between the bones, leading to stiffness and discomfort.

The second part of the problem is muscle loss. As we age, our muscles atrophy, making them weaker and less supportive of our joints. This can lead to a vicious cycle where reduced mobility leads to more inactivity, which further weakens the muscles.

Hormonal Changes

Post-menopausal women know this struggle all too well. Estrogen levels plummet, leading to increased abdominal fat. For men, testosterone levels decline, leading to muscle loss and a decrease in metabolic rate. These changes can make weight management challenging.

Lifting will be harder than it used to be, and your workout routines will need to adapt. It will take time to shed stubborn weight, and the process might be frustrating. This is part and parcel of the aging process, but it doesn't mean you can't overcome it with the right approach.

Sense and Sensibility

Then there's sensory decline. It's more than just needing reading glasses or turning up the TV volume. Balance can be compromised, making physical activity feel risky. Nearly one in three people over 65 experiences a fall each year, often due to compromised balance, as per the National Council on Aging. The hearing and vision loss that comes with age makes it harder to detect hazards, especially when exercising outdoors.

Real Barriers and Real Solutions

So, what binds all these tales together? It's the need for awareness and adaptation. The real barriers—reduced mobility, hormonal changes, sensory decline—aren't insurmountable. But they require tailored strategies. When you're informed, you can make decisions that pave the way for an active and healthy life.

In the upcoming chapters, we will delve deeper into these issues and provide practical solutions to overcome them. We will explore how cardiovascular health, muscle strength, and mental well-being are all interconnected and crucial for overall wellness.

Taking the First Step – Setting Achievable Goals

Starting on the path to getting in shape after 50 can feel like standing at the base of a mountain. It's imposing, but the journey begins with understanding where you are and where you want to go. Let's talk about how to set goals that not only seem within reach but spur you on, day after day.

Before you strap on your boots, you need a map. Self-assessment is your map. Look at your health as it stands today. Are you managing high blood pressure or diabetes? Do your knees ache after a walk around the block? These aren't just inconveniences; they are your starting point. So, take a paper and pen, and jot down where you are today. You may not like some of the things you see on this list, but don't let that discourage you. Use it as motivation for what's to come.

Here's a sample of how it might turn out -

- *Overweight*
- *High blood pressure*
- *Low energy levels*

- *Poor balance and coordination*
- *Difficulty with stairs*
- *Sedentary lifestyle*

After assessing where you are, it's time to get specific. Vague goals don't light a fire under anyone. Instead of "I want to be healthier," try "I will walk 10,000 steps a day." This is what's known as a SMART goal—Specific, Measurable, Achievable, Relevant, and Time-bound.

Let's take 'overweight' from the list above and make it into a SMART goal - "I will lose 10 pounds in three months by exercising five days a week and reducing my daily calorie intake by 500." This goal is specific, measurable, achievable (as weight loss of 1-2 pounds per week is considered healthy), relevant (it addresses the issue of being overweight that was identified in the self-assessment), and time-bound (in three months).

Or for 'sedentary lifestyle,' a SMART goal could be - "I will do 30 minutes of moderate-intensity exercise every day for one month." This goal is specific (30 minutes of exercise), measurable (moderate intensity), achievable, relevant (it addresses the issue of being sedentary), and time-bound (one month).

Life throws curveballs, and our targets need to move with them. Our bodies change, and sometimes, what worked yesterday won't work today. We need to be flexible. Consistency is key but not at the cost of burning out or causing injury. Always be open to reassessing and adjusting your goals as needed.

Best-selling author and motivational speaker, Zig Ziglar once said, "If you aim at nothing, you will hit it every time." So, set your goals and start aiming. You may not reach the peak in a day or a week or even a month, but with consistent effort and determination, you will reach it eventually.

The final piece of the puzzle is regular check-ins. Assessing progress keeps you on course and allows for necessary adjustments. Let's say you set a goal to walk 10,000 steps a day, but after two weeks, you find it's too challenging. It's okay to adjust and start with a lower step count or increase gradually. The important thing is to keep moving forward and not give up.

As you begin on this transformative journey, picture it not as a race, but as a scenic hike up a mountain. Each step is deliberate, each challenge surmountable, and the view at the summit rewarding. Our bodies change, and so should our strategies. What worked in your 30s may not be effective now. It's also about listening to your body— knowing when to push and when to rest.

Consistent effort, based on solid science and tailored to your unique needs, can yield incredible results. **Embrace this chapter of your life with enthusiasm and courage**, knowing each step, each decision, contributes to a stronger, healthier you.

CHAPTER 2

Mastering the Aging Process

"You can't help getting older, but you don't have to get old." – **George Burns**

Our bodies inevitably change. But this process isn't just a downward spiral. It's a living story filled with twists and growth. So, let's dive in and uncover what truly happens as we age and how we can navigate these changes to thrive.

Scientists have been busy decoding how and why we age. They've studied everything from worms to humans, and the consensus is clear - while we can't stop aging, we can certainly slow it down. Caloric restriction, for example, has shown promise in extending lifespan in animals by reducing metabolic processes that speed aging.

It's also worth mentioning the strides in modern medicine. From statins for cholesterol to advanced imaging techniques, today's medical landscape offers tools our grandparents could only dream of. The better we understand the aging process, the better we can prevent and treat age-related conditions. The ultimate goal isn't just longevity but health span, the period of life spent in good health.

Now, many wonder, "Is my destiny written in my genes?" The short answer is - not entirely. Genetics plays a role in how we age, but only about 20-30%. The rest? That's on you—your lifestyle choices. Choices matter – for instance, adopting a Mediterranean diet rich in vegetables, fruits, and healthy fats can add years to your life. The famed "Blue Zones"—regions where people live the longest—show that daily physical activity, a sense of purpose, and strong social communities enhance longevity.

So here's the truth - aging is a complex, multi-faceted process. Yet, with the right knowledge and approach, we can navigate it gracefully. Embrace these years with enthusiasm. Each step you take is an investment in a healthier, more vibrant future. Just like Dorothy, your choices matter.

The Different Types of Age

When we talk about aging, the questions "How old are you?" and "How old do you feel?" can lead to very different answers. Let's break down the different types of age that shape your life and health in unique ways.

Chronological Age

Chronological age is the simplest. It's the number of years you've been alive. Yet, this number doesn't necessarily dictate how well you are or how you feel. Imagine you're at a school reunion of sorts. You're surrounded by former classmates who are all the same age. But look around the room - some look like they haven't aged a day, others seem much older.

Chronological age fails to tell the whole story. Sure, it can be a predictor for health issues since risks like heart disease increase as we age. But it's not the main villain in the aging saga. The real antagonists are often lifestyle choices and medical conditions that follow us as we grow older.

Biological Age

Biological age is a measure of how your body functions and has more to do with lifestyle and genetics. Some hit their biological 60s while still in their chronological 50s, while others maintain youthful vigor well past the expected age.

Let's take two examples. First, there's Angela, my client. She's 55 years old but can run circles around most guys half her age. Then there's Astrid, who is also 55 but her sedentary lifestyle has made her feel like she's in her 70s. Despite being the same chronological age, their biological ages couldn't be more different.

Psychological Age

Then, there's psychological age, which boils down to how young or old you feel mentally.

For instance, take a lively grandfather who spends weekends hiking with his grandchildren. Although he is chronologically 80, his zest for life makes him psychologically much younger. He plans future adventures, learns new skills, and approaches life with enthusiasm. Or consider a 20-something who is constantly stressed and worried, making them feel much older than their actual age.

The theory of psychological age is rooted in the idea that one's mindset and attitude can significantly impact overall well-being. It's not just about physical health but also mental health. In our context, the psychosocial view of aging is crucial. It's a reminder that age isn't just a number, but a multifaceted concept that encompasses physical, mental, and emotional aspects.

Normal Aging

You might find yourself squinting to read the morning paper or reaching for your glasses more often. **It's presbyopia.** As we age, the lenses in our eyes thicken and lose flexibility, making it harder to focus on close objects like that book or your phone. This isn't a sign of something dire; it's simply one of those "everybody's got it" aging milestones.

Consider learning new skills. Maybe that's feeling a bit more challenging now. Increased forgetfulness, shorter attention spans, and slower learning rates are all part of the mental changes that come with age. This is **normal aging**, not to be confused with something more severe like dementia.

Now, let's talk numbers. As you get older, your blood sugar levels might rise more after a carbohydrate-heavy meal. This uptick is actually a normal part of aging. But if these levels skyrocket past a certain threshold, you're looking at diabetes. It illustrates that sometimes the difference between "normal aging" and "disorder" can be a thin line drawn by our health metrics.

There are countless other indicators of normal aging, from wrinkles and gray hair to slower metabolism and decreased bone density. To put it simply, aging isn't black-and-white. It isn't just random events strung together but a series of predictable wear-and-tear signals our bodies send us.

Healthy (Successful) Aging

But aging doesn't have to mean a downtick in your quality of life. Instead, it can be an opportunity to age in a healthy, proactive way. This process, known as "healthy aging," is all about maintaining physical and mental well-being, avoiding illnesses, and remaining active and independent.

Healthy aging isn't just about avoiding the negatives. It's about embracing the positives. Think of it as cultivating a garden. Yes, you pull the weeds, but you also plant, water, and nurture your plants so they thrive. The same goes for your health.

Creating Healthy Habits. Establishing healthy routines bit by bit—mindfully choosing nutritious foods, taking brisk walks each day, and avoiding smoking and excessive drinking. Simple changes, made consistently, can create a foundation for a healthier, more vibrant life.

The Power of Physical Activity. Engaging in regular physical activity can reduce the risk of chronic diseases like heart disease and diabetes by up to 50%. Consider a person, after a heart attack at 59, deciding to take their health into their own hands. By committing to a regimen of daily walks, strength training, and stretches, they didn't just recover—they thrived.

Mental Agility Matters Too. It's not just about the muscles and joints. Keeping your brain active is equally crucial. Learning new skills, reading, and engaging in challenging mental activities can keep the cognitive decline at bay.

Small steps towards mental agility can lead to significant rewards, enhancing your overall well-being.

Here are some numbers to chew on -

1. **Impairment Decline** - In the US, the percentage of people aged 75 to 84 who report impairments has decreased significantly in recent years.

2. **Debilitating Disorders** - There's a noted decline in the percentage of people over age 65 suffering from debilitating conditions.

3. **Longevity Growth** - The number of people living beyond 85, including centenarians, has seen a remarkable increase. This trend underscores the impact of healthy aging practices and advanced medical practices.

Living Life Fully. Healthy aging is the bridge to living your later years with fullness and vitality. While aging is inevitable, it's within our power to make those years count.

The Physiological Changes That Occur as We Age

With age comes a series of changes that can shake up the status quo. Our metabolism may slow down, our muscles lose some of their spring, and our bones may become slightly more brittle. It's all part of the package deal of growing older.

Metabolic Slowdown

You're in your early 30s, feeling invincible. Your energy levels are high, and you can eat pretty much anything without seeing a significant change in your waistline. Now let's fast forward a couple of decades. Suddenly, those same habits don't yield the same results.

As we age, our metabolism undergoes a subtle but persistent transformation. By the time we hit our 50s, our basal metabolic rate (BMR)—that's the number of calories our body burns at rest—starts to decrease. This phenomenon is largely due to a decline in muscle mass. And why does this happen? Muscles are calorie-burning machines, even when we're lounging in front of the TV. But as we grow older, muscle mass tends to wane, taking our once robust metabolism down a notch.

Let me take you through a real-life example. Meet Alice, a great friend of mine. At 35, Alice was in good shape, clocking in at a solid 140 pounds. By 55, that number crept up to 160 pounds, even though she hadn't changed her diet drastically. What gives? Alice's muscle mass had decreased by about 5%, a common figure for women her age. That meant she was burning fewer calories, even though her lifestyle hadn't changed significantly. It's like driving a car that once got amazing gas mileage but now guzzles fuel— no wonder the tank (or, in this case, the waist) is expanding!

Here's the kicker—this isn't a hopeless situation by any stretch. Though our metabolic rate slows, we have the power to mitigate these effects. Weight training and balanced nutrition can make a world of difference. The key is knowing what changes are happening so you can adapt accordingly.

Decrease in Muscle Mass

Sarcopenia—the gradual loss of muscle mass that sneaks up on us as we age. Sarcopenia doesn't just steal your muscle; it raids your strength and energy, too.

Let's dissect why this happens. First, neurons—those essential nerve cells that send signals from your brain to muscles—start to deteriorate, akin to a once-clear radio station now full of static. This fuzzy connection slows down muscle response, impacting strength and coordination.

Next, protein, the vital fuel for muscle growth. As we age, our bodies don't convert protein into energy as efficiently. It's like running on low-grade fuel. The process in our bodies is called anabolism—it's how we make and keep muscle. When this process slows down in our 30s, it doesn't necessarily register as a significant concern. But over time, these losses add up.

The famous research institute, Mayo Clinic, believes that after age 30, most people experience a loss of one-tenth of a pound of muscle per year. So by the time we're 60, we've lost about five pounds of muscle!

Changes in Body Composition

One of the most profound changes that happen is in our body composition. Specifically, there's an uninvited guest around your waistline—abdominal fat.

Abdominal fat is a red flag waving ominously over your health. As we age, fat distribution shifts more toward the belly, making this area a hotspot for health issues. More fat here isn't just uncomfortable—it's dangerous. Scientists call this type of fat "visceral fat," and it wraps around your internal organs. This increases your risk for metabolic syndrome, type 2 diabetes, and heart disease.

You see, fat gain around the abdomen isn't just about growing older. It's about your changing metabolism—the engine that runs everything from your brain to your muscles. Once our metabolism slows, like a once roaring river reduced to a gentle stream. Pair this with muscle loss (sarcopenia we discussed earlier), and you're left with a double-edged sword. Less muscle means your body burns fewer calories at rest. Your energy needs decrease, but if you eat the same, those extra calories get stored as fat.

Scientific studies bring these points home clearly. Research published in the "Journal of Clinical Endocrinology and Metabolism" shows that adults over 50 who don't exercise and maintain their diet can see their body fat increase by 30% over twenty years. It's a gradual creep, often unnoticed until significant changes have already taken place.

Body composition changes are inevitable with age, a silent evolution happening beneath your skin. Awareness is your first line of defense. Recognize these changes not as something to fear, but as essential signals your body is sending. They remind you to adapt, to listen, and to act.

Hormones - How They Shape Your Muscles!

Testosterone in Muscle Health

Testosterone is crucial for muscle protein synthesis—the process where your body builds and repairs muscle fibers. Lower testosterone means less efficient muscle repair and growth. It's like trying to fix a leaky roof with just a handful of nails. Over time, this inefficiency translates into noticeable muscle loss.

There's an enzyme called aromatase that converts testosterone into estrogen—the hormone typically associated with women. As men age, their bodies produce more aromatase, which means less testosterone and more estrogen.

Estrogen isn't all bad; it can be beneficial for bone health and preventing osteoporosis in both men and women. But when estrogen levels are too high relative to testosterone levels, it can cause a host of health issues such as decreased libido, erectile dysfunction, and increased body fat.

Estrogen in Shaping Your Health

When estrogen levels drop, it's not just one part of your body that feels the impact—everything is connected. One of the most noticeable changes is in body fat distribution. Lower estrogen levels often lead to an increase in abdominal fat.

More scientifically, these fat cells in your abdomen are active—they release hormones and other substances that can mess with your insulin sensitivity. This is why you might see your blood sugar levels creep up, even if your diet hasn't changed much.

Another silent transformation occurs in your bones and muscles. Estrogen plays a key role in maintaining bone density. Picture your bones as grand old buildings. Estrogen acts like a diligent maintenance crew, constantly repairing and adding to the structure. Without enough estrogen, the maintenance slows down, and the bones begin to weaken—a condition known as osteoporosis.

Bones become porous and fragile, raising the risk of fractures.

Estrogen also guards your muscle mass. As its levels fall, muscles lose some of their strength and mass. This isn't just about looking toned; muscles support your entire skeletal structure, protect joints, and prevent falls by stabilizing your movements.

Growth Hormone

As you inch past 50, the decline in GH begins to show its effects. Recovery after physical exertion takes longer. The bounce-back from a minor injury is slower than it used to be.

With lower GH, your body starts to struggle with maintaining muscle mass and strength. Muscle fibers don't repair as quickly, making overall physical improvement harder to achieve. This decline contributes to the subtle shifts in body composition you might see in the mirror. Maybe the waistband feels a tad snugger, or the once-toned arms seem a bit softer. This isn't just about looks—it's about health.

Growth hormone doesn't only shape your body; it supports essential functions that once operated seamlessly. Consider its role in fat metabolism. GH promotes lipolysis, breaking down fats so they can be used for energy. Reduced GH levels slow this process, making it easier to gain weight and harder to lose it. It's a significant shift, turning the effortless maintenance of earlier years into a more conscious effort.

Let's delve into my neighbor's story—Susan's. She's always been active, but now at 60, she finds climbing stairs more taxing and notices more persistent muscle soreness. She isn't eating more or exercising less, but her body composition is changing. Lower GH is the unseen hand here, reducing muscle mass and increasing fat storage. The challenge isn't just physical—it's emotional too. Understanding these changes can help, but the journey requires adjustments in lifestyle and mindset.

Growth hormone is a quiet yet powerful force in your body, especially as you age. Its decline affects everything from how you heal to how you maintain weight. This isn't just a matter of vanity—it's about staying healthy and strong. The stories of Alice and Susan are real-life examples that bring these concepts to life. Understanding GH's role helps you adapt, stay informed, and take control of your health narrative.

These hormonal changes are a domino effect. Lower growth hormone hampers our body's ability to repair muscle fibers quickly. This sluggish repair cycle means that building new muscle becomes a tough task. Fat accumulation also increases. Our metabolism slows, and the body doesn't use fats for energy as efficiently. This can lead to gradual but persistent weight gain, even if your diet and activity levels remain the same.

Taking Charge of Aging

Aging is not the enemy; it's a natural progression we all share. Each stage reveals its own set of challenges and rewards.

While we'll cover each of the different facets of tackling the aging process in later sections, let's focus on one aspect here—adaptability. To maintain vitality and enthusiasm for life, we need to be adaptable. This means understanding the changes our body is going through and taking proactive steps to counteract them.

Adaptability also means being open-minded and willing to try new things. Whether it's adjusting your workout routine or trying a new form of exercise, being adaptable allows for continued growth and improvement. It also means accepting that our bodies may change in ways we don't expect, and that's okay.

For the must haves, here's a checklist -

1. **Strength Training** - Incorporate at least 20 minutes of resistance training, three times a week.

2. **Balanced Diet** - Focus on lean proteins, healthy fats, and whole grains. Avoid processed sugars— they spike insulin, which can hamper muscle repair.

3. **Sleep** - Aim for 7-8 hours of quality sleep. This is when your body repairs muscles and balances hormones.

4. **Stay Active** - Walk, swim, or cycle regularly. Even small movements bolster heart health and hormone regulation.

5. **Monitor Progress** - Keep a journal of your workouts, diet, and how you feel. This helps spot trends and adjust as needed.

Let's also remember that aging is a journey, not a destination. It's never too late to start taking care of your body and adapting to the changes it goes through.

CHAPTER 3

The Role of Exercise in Maintaining Lean Muscle

*"Strength does not come from physical capacity. It comes from an indomitable will." - **Mahatma Gandhi***

I remember a conversation with a fine 60-year-young woman, one morning. She had just turned the decade, and despite the bright morning sun, her outlook seemed gloomy. "I feel like I am losing my strength," she said, frustration evident in her eyes. This got me thinking about how common her situation is. Many over 50 feel the same, but it's not just an inevitable part of aging.

Exercise is more than just a heart-pumping activity; it's the bedrock for maintaining muscle. **Lean muscle mass declines with age**. But this doesn't mean throwing in the towel. Think of Arnold Schwarzenegger in his 70s, still pumping iron. That's not just genetics; that's dedication and consistent training.

Our muscles are akin to a savings account. **The more you invest in them early on, the more you'll have to withdraw later.** By your 50s, it's imperative to keep those deposits coming. Personal anecdotes like the above aren't isolated. Let's take my client, Teresa, a retired teacher who started powerlifting at 65. She began with light weights due to feeling generally weak and fatigued. Within a year, she successfully deadlifted 100 pounds—an accomplishment that not only transformed her physique but also boosted her confidence and independence.

Balance and mobility are the unsung heroes here. As Dr. John Morley from Saint Louis University said, "Muscle mass is the number one biomarker of aging." Strong muscles help us move efficiently, preventing falls—a significant concern as we age.

Think of this chapter as your blueprint for action. You have the tools and examples. It's about integrating them into daily life.

Building Your Exercise Blueprint

It all starts with three things - why, how, and what. I'm sure by now, the why is clear. Now let's tackle the how and what. Let's begin with the goals.

To build lean muscle and maintain it, your workout should have two parts - strength training and cardio.

Strength Training

We've established that the aging process causes a decline in muscle mass. Strength training is all about resistance or weight-bearing exercises that work muscles against some form of resistance.

It isn't just for the young. Studies show lifting weights can boost muscle mass at any age. For example, research from the American College of Sports Medicine reveals that a mere **three sessions per week** can result in nearly two pounds of lean muscle gain in six months. This is huge!

The top recommended exercises are compound movements that use multiple muscle groups together, such as squats, deadlifts, and bench presses. But don't let these scare you; start small with bodyweight exercises if needed.

Think about it - if you start small—say, lifting five-pound dumbbells—you'll build strength over time. Just like depositing a bit of money in the bank regularly adds up. You don't need fancy equipment. **Bodyweight exercises** work wonders too. Squats, lunges, and push-ups can keep you strong if weights aren't your thing.

Cardio

But strength training alone won't cut it. Aerobic activities are your next move. Walking, cycling, and swimming are fantastic choices. These exercises improve heart health and enhance endurance. Aim for **150 minutes** of moderate aerobic activity weekly. It's easier than it sounds. A 30-minute brisk walk five days a week gets you there.

Picture yourself like an engine. The more you run it, the better it performs. Your heart, your engine, will thank you.

Let's create a plan for a typical week. Assuming the age is 56 the body weight is 160 pounds, and the goal is to maintain existing muscle mass.

- **Monday** - 30-minute strength training (using weights or bodyweight)

- **Tuesday** - 30-minute aerobic activity (brisk walking)

- **Wednesday** - Rest day

- **Thursday** - 30-minute strength training

- **Friday** - 45-minute aerobic activity (cycling)

- **Saturday** - 30-minute strength training

- **Sunday** - Rest day

Note - This is just an example. Customize your plan according to your fitness level and goals.

Flexibility and Balance Are Critical

As we age, maintaining flexibility and balance becomes crucial. Falling can lead to severe injuries, but you can prevent them. Integrating yoga or simple stretching exercises can help.

A great stretching routine that I swear by is the "pigeon pose." It stretches the hips and glutes, which are essential for balance. Just a few minutes of stretching after your workouts can make a world of difference.

Or you can consider taking a yoga or Pilates class. These are low-impact activities that focus on flexibility, balance, and building lean muscle. A balanced routine is vital.

Overloading one type of exercise won't bring the desired results.

Mind Over Matter

Finally, let's not ignore the mental game. Staying motivated is paramount. The **psychology** behind habits shows that setting small, achievable goals helps. Celebrate those small wins! Even if it's pushing out an extra rep or adding five minutes to your walk.

James Clear, the author of "Atomic Habits," recommends tracking your progress. A simple journal entry noting what you did and how it made you feel is enough. And on those days when motivation seems impossible, remind yourself why you started.

By following these steps, you'll create a sustainable and effective exercise program. In no time, you'll notice the changes. Increased muscle mass, better endurance, improved balance, and flexibility—this is the path to a healthier, more active life post-50.

Surmounting Hurdles and Staying Inspired

You're ready to get fit and strong. But let's face it, the journey isn't always straightforward. I know it can be challenging. Together, we're going to break down the barriers that often trip us up.

We're social creatures. Even in fitness, we thrive in communities. Find a group—online or in person—that shares your goals. You can even have your wife, husband, or partner join you. Support is crucial, but it's also necessary to be comfortable being alone. Letting go of self-consciousness is easier said than done, even for the most confident among us.

Think of what genuinely excites you. Is it keeping up with your grandkids? Or perhaps it's completing a charity walk. Personal goals that resonate with your life are more motivating. **Studies show** that goal-setting improves performance by up to 15%. The key is to set goals that are not only achievable but also meaningful to you.

Your body changes over time, and that's okay. Instead of seeing this as a limitation, see it as an opportunity to tune into your needs. Pain isn't gain; listen to your body. Equip yourself with knowledge. Understanding the "why" behind your workouts can be a game-changer. Dive into resources, workshops, or even online courses. Knowledge empowers you to make informed decisions. Think of it as giving yourself an edge. When you know better, you do better.

Here's the crux of it all - consistency trumps perfection. Even if you can't do a full workout, doing something is always better than doing nothing. Consistency builds habits, and habits lead to results.

Lastly, don't wait for major milestones to be celebrated. Did you manage an extra rep? Did you take an additional minute on your walk? Those are wins! Recognize and celebrate them.

You've got this. Let's make this fitness journey one that you enjoy and look forward to. Because staying fit isn't just about adding years to your life; it's about adding life to your years.

CHAPTER 4

Nutrition Essentials for Aging Well

"Let food be thy medicine and medicine be thy food."
Hippocrates

Let's talk about why what you eat matters, especially as you age. Our bodies change over time, and so should our diets. Eating the right foods can make a massive difference in how we feel, how we move, and even how we think. Here's the deal on nutrition, boiled down to what really matters.

But before that, let's get real about processed foods. They're convenient but terrible for you. Loaded with sugars, salts, and unhealthy fats, they contribute to weight gain and chronic diseases like diabetes and heart disease.

The global processed food market is growing at an alarming rate, with a projected value of $11.4 trillion by 2025. And unfortunately, seniors are among the top consumers of processed foods due to their convenience and affordability. In correlation to that, the average obesity rates among seniors have also been on the rise in recent years. Compare that to a few decades ago when the majority of seniors were lean and active, and it's clear that our modern diet has greatly contributed to this trend.

But what exactly should we be eating instead? Let's start with the basics.

Nutrient-Dense Foods

You've probably heard the saying, "You are what you eat." But ask yourself, what are you eating these days? Are your food choices helping you thrive, or are they just filling the void? When it comes to getting fit, nutrient-dense foods are your best allies. These powerhouse foods are packed with everything your body needs and nothing it doesn't. Let's break down why this matters, using real-life examples and some science-backed facts.

Think of nutrient-dense foods as the Swiss Army knife of your diet. They are loaded with vitamins, minerals, and other essential nutrients without the extra baggage of calories, fats, or sugars. Spinach, for instance, is rich in iron, which fuels your energy, and magnesium, which balances your mood. Compare that to a sugary soda—same calories, but zero benefits.

There are three main macro-nutrients - carbohydrates, proteins, and fats. While all are essential for our body's functioning, it is crucial to choose the right sources. Highly processed carbs like white bread and pasta can spike blood sugar levels and lead to weight gain over time. Instead, opt for complex carbohydrates found in whole grains, vegetables, and fruits.

Protein is your go-to nutrient. It's essential for muscle repair and maintaining a strong immune system. Think lean meats, fish, and eggs. If you prefer plant-based options, beans and lentils are excellent choices. Aim for around 0.8 grams of protein per kilogram of body weight daily. For a 70 kg person, that's about 56 grams of protein.

Likewise - berries, nuts, and colorful vegetables are anti-inflammatory powerhouses. They help combat oxidative stress, a key factor in aging. Think blueberries, they pack a punch with antioxidants. One cup of blueberries has just 85 calories but provides 24% of your daily vitamin C needs. Fiber too is vital for a healthy digestive system. Simple choices like whole grains, fruits, and veggies make a world of difference. A daily intake of 25-30 grams of fiber can keep your digestive system running smoothly.

All the above pointers lead to one thing - food diversity. The more diverse your choices, the better your chances of getting all the nutrients you need. Eat a rainbow of fruits and vegetables to get enough vitamins and minerals. Experiment with new grains like quinoa or protein-rich seeds like chia and flaxseeds.

Take a page from the Mediterranean diet, known for its heart-health benefits and longevity. This diet focuses on whole foods like fruits, vegetables, lean proteins, and healthy fats like olive oil. Research has shown that followers of the Mediterranean diet live longer, healthier lives. Incorporate elements of this diet into your daily routine for noticeable improvements.

Eating Mindfully and Why It Matters

Let's dive into a concept that could change your relationship with food - mindful eating. You're enjoying a quiet breakfast. The smell of freshly brewed coffee fills the air, and you take a moment to appreciate the vibrant colors of your fruit salad. You savor each bite, noticing the different textures and flavors. This is mindful eating - being fully present and appreciating your food.

Why does this matter? Because it transforms eating from a mindless activity to an enriching experience. Research from Harvard Health shows that mindful eating can significantly reduce overeating and help maintain a healthy weight. It encourages you to slow down, chew thoroughly, and listen to your body's hunger and fullness cues.

Here's a practical way to start -

1. When you eat, just eat. No TV, no smartphone.

2. Take small bites and chew thoroughly. Aim for 20-30 chews per bite.

3. Pay attention to the flavors, textures, and aromas of your food.

Studies prove that those who practice mindful eating are more in tune with their body's needs. They're less likely to eat out of boredom or stress. *Think of it as meditation for the stomach.*

Crafting a Balanced Diet

Here's how to build a diet that powers you through the golden years, maintaining your vitality, strength, and joy.

Proteins aren't just for bodybuilders. Think of protein as the building blocks of your body. It's crucial for maintaining muscle mass, which naturally decreases as we age. **Aim for 20-30 grams of protein per meal**. This can come from lean meats like chicken or fish, plant-based sources like beans or lentils, and dairy.

So, in an ideal day for an 80kg person, you could have -

- 3 eggs for breakfast (19g protein)
- 140g grilled chicken breast for lunch (36.4g protein)
- 1 cup of lentil soup for dinner (18g protein)
- 200ml low-fat yogurt as a snack (10g protein)

That's roughly **83 grams of protein** in one day!

Next, fats are not the enemy; they're an ally. Healthy fats support brain health, reduce inflammation, and provide long-lasting energy. Incorporate sources like **avocados, nuts, seeds, and olive oil**.

Again, an ideal day could include -

- Half an avocado with breakfast (10g fat)
- Handful of almonds for a snack (14g fat)
- Drizzle of olive oil in lunch and dinner preparations (28g fat total)

Fats have a higher calorie density than protein and carbohydrates, so be mindful of portions.

Fruits and veggies are packed with essential vitamins and minerals that keep your immune system strong and prevent chronic diseases. **Aim for at least 5 servings a day**. Think of them as colorful shields protecting your body. Bright red tomatoes, deep green spinach, and juicy blueberries—all these act as your body's frontline defenders.

Whole grains like oats, brown rice, and quinoa are equally vital. They provide sustained energy and are a great source of dietary fiber, which aids digestion.

The deal with carbs - **choose complex carbs over simple ones**. Simple carbs like white bread, pasta, and baked goods are quickly digested and can cause blood sugar spikes. Complex carbs found in whole grains, fruits, and vegetables take longer to digest, providing sustained energy without the crash.

Finally, hydration is paramount. As we age, our bodies become less efficient at retaining water. **Aim for 8 glasses per day** and choose hydrating foods like fruits and vegetables.

Creating a balanced diet doesn't have to be complicated, but it does need to be consistent. Visualize your plate - half covered in vegetables and fruits, a quarter with lean protein, and the remaining quarter with whole grains. Add a splash of healthy fat, and you're set.

This isn't about restriction; it's about abundance.

Mastering Meal Planning

Start by visualizing your week. Identify the days you have more time and those that are jam-packed. For instance, if Mondays are hectic, plan a quick, healthy meal like a quinoa salad with chicken that you can prepare on Sunday.

Dedicate one day to chopping veggies, cooking grains, and portioning out snacks. Having these elements ready eliminates the temptation of less healthy options. Ideally, plan for three main meals and two snacks per day. Your body needs fuel every 3-4 hours.

Meal planning doesn't mean you're locking yourself into rigid choices. It's about having a framework.

We eat with our eyes first. Using smaller plates can naturally reduce portion sizes. Research suggests that this simple trick can lead to consuming 22% fewer calories. Trust your hunger cues as your guide. What I recommend for one person may not work for another. For example, if you're still hungry after a meal, add more protein or healthy fats to increase satiety.

It's okay to have treats in your meal plan! The key is choosing them mindfully and enjoying them fully. Indulge in that small piece of dark chocolate or glass of wine with dinner. Depriving yourself of your favorite foods can lead to binge eating and feelings of guilt.

A pro tip - Use a grocery list! This prevents impulsive buys, saves you time and money, and keeps you on track with your meal plan.

Start small. Adapt as needed. Overcomplicating your plan can lead to burnout. It's like building a house, laying one brick at a time ensures the foundation is strong.

Mastering Cravings

Let's face it - cravings can derail even the most well-laid dietary plans. But there's good news—taking control of your cravings doesn't have to feel like a battle.

Cravings often originate from nutritional deficiencies, stress, or simply habits formed over time. For example, craving salty snacks might mean a lack of minerals like potassium or magnesium, whereas a longing for sweets could be your body asking for more magnesium or chromium.

To outsmart your cravings, here's what you can do -

- *Increase your intake of nutrient-dense foods like fruits, vegetables, and whole grains. This will help address any underlying deficiencies.*

- *Prioritize self-care to reduce stress levels. Incorporate activities like yoga or meditation into your daily routine.*

- *Identify alternative habits that satisfy the same emotional need as cravings. For instance, if you crave chocolate when feeling sad, try calling a friend or going for a walk instead.*

Cravings don't have to control you. You have the power to make mindful choices and nourish your body in a way that makes you feel good. And remember, it's all about balance and moderation. Enjoying your favorite treats in moderation is part of a healthy lifestyle.

These aren't just tips; they're stepping stones to a healthier you. Integrate them one at a time and see how they fit. Making informed choices every day adds up, transforming your health and well-being.

CHAPTER 5

Superfoods and Supplements for Aging Gracefully

"To give anything less than your best is to sacrifice the gift."
Steve Prefontaine

Let's talk about aging gracefully. It's not just about adding years to your life but adding life to your years. Enter superfoods and supplements—the unsung heroes that can help you stay vibrant and healthy.

Imagine superfoods as little power-packed gems. They're nutrient-rich and bring immense benefits to your health. When we say "superfoods," think of berries loaded with antioxidants, like blueberries or strawberries. These aren't just tasty snacks. They fight off free radicals, helping to reduce inflammation and support brain health.

Understanding these superfoods and supplements is only half the battle. Incorporating them into your daily life is where the magic happens. Start small. Add a handful of nuts to your breakfast or a teaspoon of chia seeds to your smoothie. You don't have to transform your entire diet overnight, but small changes can yield big results. Don't worry, we'll dive into the specific superfoods and supplements that can help you age gracefully in this chapter.

In a nutshell, superfoods and supplements aren't magic beans, but they are powerful allies. They support your journey to stay active, healthy, and vibrant—no matter your age.

The Power of Superfoods

Incorporating superfoods into your diet can have dramatic health benefits. But what makes these foods so powerful? Let's break it down.

Imagine you're a builder—your body needs high-quality materials to construct a strong, durable structure. **Superfoods** are those materials. They provide essential nutrients that are vital for maintaining and enhancing your health. Instead of indulging in empty calories, think of these foods as nutrient-dense options that fuel your longevity.

Berries like blueberries, strawberries, and blackberries are loaded with antioxidants. Antioxidants are compounds that prevent or delay cell damage. For example, a handful of blueberries daily can significantly reduce oxidative stress.

Oxidative stress is a balance of free radicals (unstable molecules) and antioxidants in your body. When there's an imbalance, free radicals can damage cells and lead to diseases related to aging. Take heart conditions, for example; free radicals can damage vital heart tissues and increase the risk of diseases like atherosclerosis. Berries also contain anthocyanins—a type of antioxidant that has been linked to improved brain function and reduced inflammation. So, not just a tasty treat, but also a powerful ally in the aging process.

Similarly, spinach, kale, and swiss chard aren't just for salads. They are packed with vitamins A, C, and K, as well as calcium and fiber. A serving a day can make a difference—think of it as reinforcing your body's defenses.

Fatty fish such as salmon and sardines are rich in Omega-3 fatty acids. These essential fats reduce inflammation and improve heart health. The American Heart Association notes that around two servings of fatty fish per week can lower the risk of heart attacks by nearly 20%. That's as straightforward as it gets—simple, tangible benefits for your heart.

Turmeric has been used for centuries for its healing properties. Curcumin, the active compound in turmeric, has strong anti-inflammatory effects. Ask the Chinese and Indians, and they'll tell you it's a traditional remedy for many ailments. Try adding a pinch to your stir-fries or soups for an extra health boost.

Changing your diet doesn't have to be daunting. Start with small, manageable steps -

1. Add a handful of nuts to your breakfast.

2. Sprinkle chia seeds on your smoothie.

3. Choose a superfood snack like berries instead of processed sweets.

Remember, it's about making sustainable changes. Each small step is a move toward a healthier, more vibrant life.

For a more detailed overview, let's break it down into action-packed, easy-to-follow steps.

Imagine a typical morning - You groggily reach for your cup of coffee, the aroma tempting yet devoid of nutrients. Now, what if you swap that routine with a vibrant smoothie? A mix of **berries** (rich in antioxidants), a **banana** (loaded with potassium and magnesium), and a handful of **spinach** (packed with vitamins A, C, K, and iron). Blend these with a scoop of **protein powder**. Not only is it tasty, but it's a powerhouse of nutrients to kickstart your day.

Salads aren't just rabbit food. Think of them as a blank canvas. A simple base of **leafy greens** like kale or spinach can be transformed. Add colorful vegetables like **cherry tomatoes** and **cucumbers**. Sprinkle a handful of **nuts** and **seeds**, which are high in good fats. For protein, consider grilled **salmon** or a sprinkle of **quinoa**. These ingredients don't just add flavor; they provide essential nutrients to keep you energized.

We all know that mid-afternoon slump. Instead of reaching for a bag of chips, keep snacks like **almonds** or **chia seeds** within reach. They are not only crunchy and satisfying but also a great source of omega-3 fatty acids and fiber. Speaking from experience, swapping out processed snacks for nutrient-dense options can make a noticeable difference in your energy levels and mental clarity.

Dinner is where you can get creative. How about a **quinoa bowl** with roasted vegetables and a side of **grilled chicken**? Quinoa is a complete protein, meaning it contains all nine essential amino acids. It's a fantastic alternative to pasta or rice. Pair it with **avocado**, which offers healthy fats that keep your heart happy. For a burst of flavor, a splash of **lemon juice** or a sprinkle of **herbs** can elevate the entire dish.

Superfoods aren't a magic bullet, but they are an essential part of a well-rounded diet. They can help you manage your weight, keep your heart ticking strongly, and even boost your mood. So, here's a simple task - make one change today. Maybe it's that morning smoothie or a handful of almonds. Embrace these superfoods and watch as your energy, mood, and health improve. Your future self will thank you.

To sum up, superfoods are packed with vitamins, minerals, antioxidants, and other beneficial compounds that help protect your body from disease and support healthy aging. Let's move on to supplements—the not-so-secret weapon in the aging game.

Maximize Your Health with the Right Supplements

Supplements can be the missing piece in our health puzzle, especially as we age. Let's break it down and make it as simple as possible, just like building a fort with strong and sturdy blocks.

One of the key supplements everyone should consider is **Vitamin D**. Our skin makes Vitamin D when exposed to sunlight, but as we age, our skin's ability to produce Vitamin D diminishes. According to the National Institutes of Health (NIH), a daily supplement can lower the risk of osteoporosis by up to 30%.

People living above the 37th parallel North, which is approximately the latitude of San Francisco, may struggle to produce enough Vitamin D in winter. That's a lot of people! Make sure to talk to your doctor about supplementing if you live in colder climates.

Next on the list is **Calcium**. As we get older, our bones naturally become less dense, increasing the risk of fractures. For post-menopausal women, this is particularly crucial. Regular intake of Calcium can help maintain bone strength. Imagine your bones as the supporting walls of our fort; without enough calcium, these walls can weaken.

You can get calcium from foods like dairy products, leafy greens, and fortified cereals. But if you're not getting enough through your diet, supplements can help fill the gap.

Other minerals are also essential to our health, such as **Magnesium** and **Potassium**. Magnesium is crucial for healthy nerve and muscle function, while potassium helps regulate blood pressure and prevent kidney stones. While you can get these minerals from foods like nuts, seeds, legumes, and leafy greens, supplements can help ensure you're getting enough.

Remember, supplements are not a substitute for a healthy diet but rather a way to fill in the gaps. Start with what matters most to you. If bone health is a worry, prioritize Vitamin D and Calcium. If you're concerned about heart health, focus on Omega-3s. By making informed choices and acting on them, you're investing in your health and longevity.

Take these insights to heart and make informed decisions that benefit your long-term wellness. It's all about small, smart choices that lead to a healthier, happier life.

Supplements and Medications

When it comes to supplements and medications, it's crucial to tread carefully. Mixing these can sometimes cause unexpected results. Let's talk about why and how you can stay safe.

Take my client, Denise, a vibrant 58-year-old retiree who loves her morning walks. She decided to add a fish oil supplement for heart health. What she didn't realize is that fish oil can thin the blood. Since Denise was also taking an aspirin daily, this combination increased her risk of bleeding. What seemed harmless posed a significant risk.

Why does this happen? It's simple. Supplements contain active ingredients that can interact with medications. This doesn't mean you should avoid all supplements, but you should understand potential interactions.

Key Interactions to Watch For

1. **Blood Thinners and Omega-3 Fatty Acids** - If you're on blood thinners like warfarin, adding an omega-3 supplement could heighten your bleeding risk. Always consult your doctor.

2. **Calcium and Antibiotics** - Calcium can interfere with the absorption of certain antibiotics, reducing their effectiveness. Separate your calcium and antibiotic doses by a few hours to avoid this.

3. **St. John's Wort and Antidepressants** - This herbal remedy is popular for managing mild depression. However, it can dangerously interact with prescription antidepressants, often leading to serotonin syndrome – a potentially life-threatening condition.

Dr. Jane Smith, a renowned geriatrician, often tells her patients, *"Think of your body as a finely tuned engine. Each supplement or medication is a component. If you add something new, it needs to fit perfectly with what's already there."*

Choosing the Right Supplements

With so many options out there, how do you know which ones are worth your time and money? Trust me, I'm here to break this down for you. Think of selecting supplements like choosing ingredients for your favorite recipe - you want only the best quality to make it memorable and effective. Here's how you can ensure you're picking high-quality supplements.

First, always look for third-party testing. Imagine you're buying a car. Would you purchase one without a safety test? Probably not. The same logic applies here. Brands like USP or NSF International test supplements rigorously to ensure they provide exactly what they promise—no more, no less. This isn't just a stamp on a bottle; it's your safety net.

Next, buy from reputable manufacturers. Companies known for their stringent quality checks and research-backed products are your best bet. Ever heard of Thorne or Pure Encapsulations? These brands invest heavily in their research and manufacturing processes to ensure you get top-notch products. It's like buying furniture from IKEA versus a random brand—you know what to expect from IKEA, right?

Athletic Greens is another brand that stands out in the world of supplements. They use high-quality, whole-food ingredients and have a comprehensive testing process to ensure each batch meets their strict standards. Plus, they're transparent about their sourcing and production methods.

One-size-fits-all doesn't work here. Tailor your supplement choices to your health needs. Suppose your bone health is a concern, look for vitamin D and calcium combinations. Dr. Andrew Weil, a pioneer in integrative medicine, often emphasizes the value of **personalized nutrition**. He isn't swayed by trends; instead, he advocates for choices based on individual conditions and blood tests.

So what should you do next? Keep it simple. Start small -

1. **Consult your healthcare provider** before starting any new supplement. They know your medical history and can help you avoid dangerous interactions.

2. **Stay informed**. Websites like NIH provide solid, updated info on supplement interactions.

3. **Track your intake**. Maintain a simple log of what you're taking and how you feel. This can provide valuable feedback for both you and your healthcare provider.

By taking these steps, you're not just adding pills to your routine; you're making informed decisions about your health. Remember, you're in control. Make choices that empower you to live your best life.

We are all going to age, but it's up to us how we do it. Supplements and superfoods can help, but they're only a part of the puzzle.

CHAPTER 6

Protein and Its Requirements for Optimal Health

"All great achievements require time."
Maya Angelou

I have been harping on the importance of protein in our diet throughout this book and for good reason. It's the essential nutrient that builds and repairs, that fuels and sustains. Especially as we age, protein's role becomes even more critical. It's not just about muscles – protein impacts everything from our immune system to our energy levels.

Visualize protein as the bricks and mortar of your house. Each meal rich in protein adds another layer of strength and resilience to your body's structure. Without it, your body's framework begins to weaken, affecting muscle strength, bone density, and overall health.

Consider this - Researchers from McMaster University found that older adults who consumed 1.5 grams of protein per kilogram of body weight per day saw significant improvements in muscle mass and strength. That's about 102 grams of protein daily for someone weighing 150 pounds. It's achievable with mindful eating.

You might worry that increasing protein means high-calorie intake. Not necessarily. Lean meats, low-fat dairy, and plant-based proteins offer low-calorie, high-protein options.

So here's the deal - in this chapter, we're going to dive deeper into the importance of protein for optimal health and discuss the recommended daily intake, sources of protein, and how to incorporate more protein into your diet.

Why Protein is Essential for Optimal Health

Let's start with metabolism. Protein isn't just for muscles. It boosts metabolism too. It takes more energy to digest protein than fats or carbs. That means more calories burned just by eating! This is a big win as our metabolism slows with age. Eating protein helps manage weight without extra effort.

To illustrate further the role of protein in metabolism, one study found that participants who consumed a high-protein diet had an 80-100% higher metabolism than those on a low-protein diet. This is because protein has a more significant thermic effect compared to carbs and fats, meaning it takes more energy to process and digest.

Then there's tissue repair. Proteins are essential for this. They build and fix tissues, helping you recover faster from injuries. They also support the immune system by generating antibodies. This is super important, especially as our immune systems weaken with age.

The science behind it - Proteins are made up of amino acids, and our bodies need 20 different types to function. Of these 20, nine are considered essential because our bodies cannot produce them on their own – we must obtain them through food sources. These essential amino acids play a crucial role in everything from muscle growth to neurotransmitter production.

The story doesn't end with muscle and metabolism. Proteins are behind many hormones and enzymes that keep our bodies ticking. These proteins are crucial for digestion and regulating hormones. Ensuring you get enough protein means these processes run smoothly, keeping you feeling your best.

Determining Individual Protein Needs

Okay, let's talk numbers. You might be wondering, "How much protein do I need?" A typical adult needs about 0.8 grams of protein per kilogram of body weight. For someone over 50, aim higher. Research suggests that 1.2 to 2.0 grams per kilogram is ideal.

For context, if you weigh 150 pounds (68 kilograms), that's about 82 to 136 grams of protein daily.

Imagine a typical meal - a grilled chicken breast (31 grams), a cup of Greek yogurt (20 grams), and half a cup of lentils (9 grams). You've got 60 grams right there. Add a smoothie with whey protein (20 grams), and you're covered.

If you're one of those who likes things down to the last decimal, here's the formula - 0.8 grams of protein per kilogram of body weight x your weight in kilograms. If pounds are all you know, divide your weight in pounds by 2.2 to get your weight in kilograms.

Your activity level matters too. *Are you lifting weights? Running?* You'll need more protein to help your muscles recover and grow. Think of protein as the bricks for building a strong, healthy house – your body. Without enough bricks, the house can't stand strong.

Chronic conditions can affect your needs too. Diabetes, arthritis, or recovering from surgery? Higher protein can help with recovery and managing these conditions. Dr. Ruth Heidrich, an Ironman triathlete, after a breast cancer diagnosis at 47, switched to a plant-based diet rich in protein. Even in her 80s, she's the epitome of health and strength. Her story shows the remarkable impact of a good protein diet.

It's one thing to know your target. It's another to hit it daily. Here are practical tips -

- **Plan Ahead** - Prep your meals. Include a variety of protein sources like chicken, fish, eggs, beans, and nuts.

- **Snack Smart** - Reach for high-protein snacks like Greek yogurt or a handful of almonds.

- **Balance Your Plate** - Make sure each meal has a good protein source.

- **Stay Informed** - Use food apps to track your protein intake.

A diet rich in diverse protein sources will keep you strong and vibrant. Refer often to your plan and adjust as needed.

Finding the Best Protein Sources

When it comes to protein, not all sources are made equal. Let's dig into the high-quality options that will support your health goals in practical, tasty, and sustainable ways. Your protein choices matter, and I'll show you why and how with real-life insights.

Animal-Based Protein Sources

1. **Lean Meats** - Think of chicken, turkey, and lean cuts of beef. They're rich in protein and pack essential amino acids that your body needs. For example, a 3-ounce chicken breast provides about 26 grams of protein. Stick to lean cuts; they have less fat and more nutrients.

2. **Fish and Seafood** - Opt for salmon, tuna, or mackerel. These fish aren't just high in protein – they are rich in omega-3 fatty acids, which are great for heart health. A six-ounce serving of salmon offers around 40 grams of protein along with omega-3s.

3. **Dairy Products** - Milk, yogurt, and cheese are great for protein and calcium. Greek yogurt, for instance, delivers about 15 grams of protein per serving. Choose low-fat options to keep your saturated fat intake in check.

4. **Eggs** - Eggs are a powerhouse of nutrients. With all nine essential amino acids, they're a complete protein. One egg has around 6 grams of protein. They're versatile and nutrient-rich.

Plant-Based Protein Sources

1. **Legumes** - Beans, lentils, chickpeas – these are not only loaded with protein but also high in fiber, vitamins, and minerals. One cup of cooked lentils provides 18 grams of protein. They're filling and perfect for soups or stews.

2. **Nuts and Seeds** - Almonds, walnuts, chia seeds, and flax seeds come packed with protein and healthy fats. A handful of almonds has about 6 grams of protein. They make for a quick, nutritious snack.

3. **Tofu and Tempeh** - These soy products are excellent meat alternatives, each bringing complete protein to the table. Choose organic to avoid genetically modified organisms (GMOs). A cup of tofu offers approximately 20 grams of protein.

4. **Whole Grains** - Quinoa, brown rice, and oats are moderate in protein but also excellent sources of fiber and essential minerals. A cup of cooked

quinoa has about 8 grams of protein. They're perfect for salads or as side dishes.

Making Protein a Daily Habit

But how do you make sure you're getting enough protein each day? Let's break it down in a way that fits easily into your routine.

Mornings can be hectic. But starting your day with protein doesn't have to be. Instead of reaching for a sugary cereal, try Greek yogurt topped with nuts and berries. It's quick, delicious, and packs in about 20 grams of protein. Eggs are another powerhouse. Scramble two eggs with spinach for a nutritious boost totaling around 12 grams. Even a simple protein smoothie with almond milk and a scoop of protein powder gets you around 25 grams.

Lunch is a prime opportunity to add lean proteins into your diet. How about a grilled chicken salad? It's easy to prepare and rich in nutrients. A single grilled chicken breast offers about 30 grams of protein. Not a fan of chicken? Opt for a can of tuna instead—it provides around 40 grams. Pair it with a quinoa side dish. Quinoa is not just a grain; it's a complete protein with about 8 grams per cup.

For dinner, it's hard to go wrong with fish. Salmon is an excellent choice. A six-ounce serving provides approximately 40 grams of protein and is loaded with heart-healthy omega-3s. Serve it with a side of lentils for an extra 18 grams. Not in the mood for fish? Swap it out for a lean cut of beef, like sirloin, which offers 46 grams of protein in a six-ounce portion.

Snacks can be a sneaky way to up your protein intake without even noticing. A handful of almonds has about 6 grams of protein and can easily be part of your daily routine. Hummus is another great option. Pair it with raw veggies for a tasty, nutrient-dense snack that adds roughly 12 grams of protein per serving.

Let's talk about timing and strategy for including protein in your diet. Starting off, **pre-workout protein** is like fueling up before a long drive. You wouldn't drive on empty, right? Have a little protein 30-60 minutes before you exercise. Think Greek yogurt parfait or a quick protein smoothie. This gives you the energy to push harder and perform better.

Next up, **post-workout protein** is crucial. It's like when you finally get home and need a good meal. Your muscles need recovery. Aim to eat within 30-60 minutes after exercising to maximize muscle repair. A simple turkey and avocado wrap, a chicken quinoa bowl, or a protein shake can make a huge difference.

Spread out your intake throughout the day. This doesn't mean obsessing over numbers. Add protein to each meal and snack. It'll keep you full longer and supply a steady stream of amino acids to your muscles. Just try to be consistent. Eggs at breakfast, chicken at lunch, fish at dinner, and almonds for a snack cover your bases without turning every meal into a science experiment.

Protein Supplementation

We've covered the importance of protein for overall health, especially as we age. Now, let's tackle how supplements can play a role in your diet. This section will break down the essentials. Think of it as your roadmap to making smart choices with supplements.

Whey protein is a game-changer. Do you remember the days of mixing protein powders that tasted like chalk? Those days are long gone. Whey protein is not only beneficial but delicious and versatile. For those who struggle to get enough protein through food alone, whey supplements can be a lifesaver. Mix it with milk, toss it into your morning oatmeal, or blend it into a smoothie. In terms of numbers, aim for about 20-30 grams of whey protein post-workout to aid muscle recovery.

Then there's collagen. Beyond its reputation as a skin anti-ager, collagen does wonders for joint health and muscle recovery. Collagen production declines as we age, leading to stiffer joints and less elasticity in the skin. To counteract this, adding collagen supplements can be a practical approach. Just mix it into your coffee or even soups.

Lastly, branched-chain amino acids (BCAAs), especially leucine, play a significant role. BCAAs are known to stimulate muscle protein synthesis. This isn't just bro-science talk; it's backed by researchers. Consider taking BCAAs if you find that muscle soreness slows you down.

Especially before or during your workout, they can make a noticeable difference.

Before diving into this supplement frenzy, there are a few ground rules. Consult with your healthcare provider or a registered dietitian. Understand what you need based on your unique health status. Remember, supplements aren't replacements for real food. They fill gaps, not entire nutritional voids. Keep track of what you're taking and adjust it as needed.

Think of supplements as the co-star in your health journey. They support but shouldn't overshadow the main show—whole foods. Combining real food with smart supplement choices sets you up for success. Picture your health journey as a well-directed movie. You're the director calling the shots, and these tips are your script for a blockbuster performance. Whether you're looking to improve joint health or bounce back faster after workouts, these strategies are your go-to guide.

If there's one thing in your diet that you should never skimp on, it's protein. The benefits of a high-protein diet, both for overall health and fitness goals, are undeniable. So, keep all these tips in mind and start incorporating more protein into your diet. Your body will thank you!

CHAPTER 7

Recipe Makeovers for Healthier Eating

"The first wealth is health."
Ralph Waldo Emerson

Cooking healthy doesn't mean giving up your favorite foods. It's about tweaking those beloved recipes to make them work for you. Imagine enjoying a delicious spaghetti Bolognese that's not only tasty but also good for your heart. Recipe makeovers can help you achieve that balance. In this chapter, we'll show you how.

In a world where quick often means unhealthy, knowing how to modify your favorite dishes to be healthier is a game-changer. Let's dive into why and how these changes matter.

Traditional recipes can be calorie-laden, thanks to ingredients like heavy creams and refined sugars. For instance, swapping out regular sour cream for Greek yogurt can cut calories while boosting protein. It's a small change but adds up over time. Imagine saving 100 calories per meal, which could mean losing up to 10 pounds a year without feeling deprived.

Healthier recipe versions help manage your weight by providing satisfying, nutrient-rich meals. High-fiber foods like lentils or chickpeas are excellent substitutes for meat. They not only lower your calorie intake but also promote a feeling of fullness.

Every small change contributes to a healthier lifestyle. With these new strategies, you can enjoy your favorite foods while taking care of your body. Next, we'll delve into the practical steps to start reworking those recipes. Stick with us, and you'll see how easy and rewarding it is to make healthier choices every day.

Exploring New Flavors While Staying Healthy

Healthy eating doesn't mean bland or boring. Think of it as adding spices to your life. Trying new ingredients and techniques can make mealtime exciting. Remember when you first tried quinoa? It was different, but now it's a staple. That's the joy of food exploration.

Let's discuss some practical, tasty changes. Take mashed potatoes. They are delicious but can be heavy. Swap half the potatoes with cauliflower. You still get the creamy texture with half the calories and more vitamins. Another example is French fries. Instead, cut sweet potatoes into strips, toss them in olive oil and bake. Delicious with a fraction of the fat.

We're not asking you to give up your favorites. Small tweaks make a big difference. Using Greek yogurt instead of sour cream adds protein and reduces fat. Mix it into your taco night routine. Or think about spaghetti Bolognese. Switching from regular pasta to whole-grain increases fiber and keeps you full longer. Even celebrity chef Jamie Oliver swears by these changes.

It's about consistency. Imagine saving just 50 calories every dinner. Over a month, that's 1,500 calories saved. Over a year, you could lose 5 pounds without sacrificing flavor. Keep an open mind. New foods can be fun and beneficial. Before dismissing kale, try it in a smoothie with fruits. You'd be surprised how little you taste it, but the health benefits are immense.

Transforming Your Favorite Recipes for Health and Flavor

Let's dive straight in. Making healthier versions of your beloved recipes doesn't have to be complicated. It's all about intelligent swaps and mindful choices.

Start by swapping high-calorie ingredients for more nutritious options. Replace refined grains with whole grains like brown rice or quinoa. This change increases fiber, which helps with digestion and keeps you full longer. *Did you know* that switching from white pasta to whole grain can cut down on blood sugar spikes? It's true and it's a small step with a significant impact.

Adding more vegetables is a game-changer. Vegetables are high in nutrients and low in calories. Let's take pasta, for example. Spiralize zucchini or thinly slice bell peppers.

You'll add volume and nutrients without extra calories. This is like using more mint leaves to bulk up a drink without adding calories—except it's a meal.

Consider adding vegetables to unexpected places for moisture and nutrients. Carrots or zucchini in your muffins or meatballs can be a delightful surprise. More and more studies show that vegetables can drastically reduce the risk of chronic diseases. For instance, a Harvard study notes that each daily serving of leafy greens can lower heart disease risk by 11%.

Spices are your best friends. Instead of using extra salt or high-calorie sauces, reach for your spice cabinet. Herbs, spices, citrus zest, and vinegar can make your dishes more exciting. *Think of how the Mediterranean diet*—praised for heart health—relies heavily on spices and herbs. Not only does this tweak reduce your sodium intake, but it also adds antioxidants.

Finally, adopt healthier cooking methods. Baking, grilling, steaming, or sautéing with minimal oil are excellent options. These techniques help maintain the nutrients in your food and reduce unhealthy fats. Thought leaders like nutritionist *Dr. Michael Greger* advocate these methods, as they help preserve the natural benefits of your ingredients.

Delicious and Satisfying Recipes for Every Meal

Whipping up tasty and satisfying meals is the secret sauce to sticking with a healthy eating plan. Here are some nutritious recipes for breakfast, lunch, and dinner that are low in calories but high in nutritional value—bon appétit without the guilt!

Tropical Protein Smoothie

- Prep Time - 10 mins
- Total time - 10 mins
- Meal type - Breakfast, Lunch, Snack, Slide.

Serving - 1

Ingredients

- *1 serving Vanilla Protein Powder, plant-based or whey (or equivalent of 20 grams protein)*
- *1/2 cup pineapple, fresh, chopped (or frozen)*
- *1 1/2 cups almond milk, unsweetened*
- *1/3 cup kale, spines removed and chopped*
- *1 tsp coconut oil, melted*
- *1/2 lime, juiced*

Instructions

- ☐ *Chop Pineapple [or used frozen chunks]*
- ☐ *Remove spines from kale and Chop leaves*
- ☐ *Place all ingredients in a high-speed blender and process until smooth.*

Butter Chip Ice Cream with Cottage Cheese

- Prep Time - 10 mins
- Total time - 4 hrs
- Meal type - Breakfast, Lunch, Snack

Serving - 2

Ingredients

- *2 cups cottage cheese, whole - milk*
- *1/4 cup maple syrup*
- *1/2 cup peanut butter powder*
- *2 Tbsp chocolate Chips, semi-sweet*

Instructions

- ☐ *Add cottage cheese, maple syrup, and peanut butter powder to a food processor. process until smooth and creamy*
- ☐ *Pulse in chocolate chips*
- ☐ *Pour into a loaf pan and freeze for 4 hours*
- ☐ *Remove and let rest to soften for about 10 minutes before serving.*

Pumpkin Cheesecake Chia Pudding

- Prep Time - 5 mins
- Total time - 4 hours
- Meal type - Breakfast, Snack

Serving – 2

Ingredients

- *1/2 cup pumpkin puree, canned*
- *¾ cup cottage cheese*
- *½ tsp vanilla extract*
- *2 Tbsp maple syrup*
- *¼ cup chia seeds*
- *2 Tbsp flax meal*
- *1 cup almond milk, unsweetened (or other milk of choice)*
- *1 ½ tsp pumpkin pie spice*
- *2 Tbsp Pumpkin seeds*

Instructions

- ☐ *Add all ingredients, except pumpkin seeds, to a blender and process until smooth.*
- ☐ *Top with pumpkin seeds.*
- ☐ *Place in a covered container or mason jars and refrigerate for at least 4 hours or overnight.*

Blueberry Cheesecake Smoothie

- Prep Time - 5 mins
- Total time - 7 mins
- Meal type - Breakfast, Snack.

Serving – 4

Ingredients

- *1 cup low-fat cottage cheese*
- *1 tsp cinnamon*
- *One medium banana*
- *1 ½ cups blueberries*
- *1 cup milk or milk of choice*
- *One graham cracker crumbled (4 squares)*

Instructions

- ☐ *Cover all ingredients except the graham cracker in a blender container. Blend on High for about 30 or 45 seconds or until smooth.*
- ☐ *Place graham crackers on the bottom of each serving glass. Pour the smoothie mixture over the cracker and enjoy!*

Ginger Berry Smoothie

- Prep Time - 5 mins
- Total time - 5 mins
- Meal type - Breakfast, Snack.

Serving – 2

Ingredients

- *½ cup plain Greek yogurt*
- *One banana, frozen*

- *1 ½ cups mixed berries*
- *1 inch ginger, peeled and chopped*
- *1 cup almond milk, unsweetened*
- *1 Tbsp almond butter*

Instructions

- ☐ *Place all the ingredients in a blender and puree on the high until smooth.*
- ☐ *Add almond milk that is too thin if the mixture is too thick to drink with a straw.*

Pineapple Cheesecake Chia Pudding

- Prep Time - 5 mins
- Total time - 4 hrs
- Meal type - Breakfast, Snack

Serving - 2

Ingredients

- *1 cup pineapple, chopped*
- *½ cup cottage cheese*
- *4 Tbsp Greek yogurts, plain, low-fat*
- *¼ tsp vanilla extract*
- *1 Tbsp maple syrup*
- *¼ cup chia seeds*
- *1 cup almond milk, unsweetened*

Instructions

- ☐ *Chop Pineapple. Reserve a few tablespoons for garnish*
- ☐ *Add all ingredients to a blender and process until smooth.*

☐ *Place in a covered container or mason jars and refrigerate for at least 4 hours or overnight.*

Chocolate Fudge Smoothie

- Prep Time - 10 mins
- Total time - 10 mins
- Meal type - Breakfast, Snack, Side.

Serving - 2

Ingredients

- *1 cup coconut milk, canned*
- *1 cup zucchini, chopped and frozen*
- *¼ cup cocoa powder, unsweetened*
- *Two Medjool dates, pitted and chopped*
- *1 Tbsp almond butter*
- *Salt, pinch*
- *1/2 cup water (or more if needed)*

Instructions

☐ *Chop and freeze zucchini*

☐ *Add all ingredients to a blender and process until smooth and creamy.*

☐ *Add more water as needed to process.*

Green Detox Smoothie

- Prep Time - 5 mins
- Total time - 5 mins
- Meal type - Breakfast, Lunch, Snack, Side.

Serving - 1

Ingredients

- *1 cup romaine lettuce, chopped*
- *1/2 cup pineapple, chopped*
- *One ginger, peeled and chopped (for 1 Tbs)*
- *1 cup cucumber, peeled and chopped*
- *2 cups water*
- *Two kiwis, peeled and chopped*
- *2 Tbsp parsley, fresh, chopped*
- *¼ avocado*
- *Stevia, to taste (optional)*

Instructions

- ☐ *Chop romaine and pineapple.*
- ☐ *Peel and chop ginger, cucumber, and kiwis*
- ☐ *Remove flesh from 1/4 avocado.*
- ☐ *Add ingredients to the blender and process until smooth. Add more water as needed.*

Blueberry Chocolate Detox Smoothie

- Prep Time - 5 mins
- Total time - 5mins
- Meal type - Breakfast

Serving – 2

Ingredients

- *2 cups blueberries, frozen*
- *2 cups spinach, baby*
- *One banana*
- *2 Tbsp chia seeds*
- *2 cups almond milk, unsweetened or milk of choice*
- *2 Tbsp cocoa powder, unsweetened*

Instructions

- ☐ *Place all ingredients in a blender and process until smooth.*

PBJ Smoothie

- Prep Time - 5 mins
- Total time - 5 mins
- Meal type - Breakfast, Snack

Serving – 1

Ingredients

- *½ cup strawberries, frozen*
- *½ cup raspberries, frozen*
- *½ banana, chopped and frozen*
- *1 cup almond milk, unsweetened*
- *2 Tbsp peanut butter powder*
- *1 Tbsp chia seeds*
- *1 tsp vanilla*
- *One date, pitted and chopped (maple syrup)*
- *¼ cup spinach, frozen*

Instructions

- ☐ *Place all ingredients in a high-speed blender and process until smooth.*

Tropical Green Smoothie

- Prep Time - 10 mins
- Total time - 10 mins
- Meal type - Breakfast, Snack.

Serving - 1

Ingredients

- *½ Banana, frozen fresh*
- *½ cup pineapple, frozen*
- *½ Avocado*
- *½ cup kale, frozen (or spinach)*
- *1 Tbsp chia seeds*

- *Eight cashews, raw*
- *1 cup almond milk, unsweetened (or milk of choice)*

Instructions

- ☐ *Chop fruits*
- ☐ *Measure ingredients*
- ☐ *Place all ingredients in a high-speed blender and process until smooth.*
- ☐ *Add water for a thinner consistency or add ice for a thicker consistency.*

Meal Preparation for Busy Lifestyles

Maintaining a healthy eating routine can be challenging, especially when life gets busy. But it's possible with a bit of planning and some smart strategies.

Let's start with the basics. **Choose simple, versatile recipes.** Look for dishes that can easily be tweaked or reused. For instance, cook a big batch of grilled chicken. Tonight, it's for dinner with veggies. Tomorrow, it's in a salad or sandwich. The key here is flexibility. If you're tired of chicken, switch it out for turkey or tofu.

Next, **batch cooking and prepping ingredients** is a real time-saver. Spend an hour on Sunday night chopping veggies or cooking grains. Store them in containers, ready to be tossed together during the hectic weekdays. Psychologically, this act of prepping can also reduce weekday stress. You're less likely to reach for unhealthy snacks when healthy meals are just a few steps away.

Investing in the right kitchen tools can make all the difference. An instant pot can become your best friend. Throw in your ingredients in the morning, set it, and come home to a hot, healthy meal. On this note, think of your appliances as your cooking assistants. They can save you a ton of hands-on time.

Think of meal prepping like laying the foundation for a sturdy house. Every ingredient prepped and every meal planned strengthens the structure. In turn, this supports you in living a healthier, more balanced life. It's not about perfection, but about making consistent, incremental improvements. With these strategies, you're on your way to achieving the best shape of your life—one meal at a time.

Making the most of your healthy meals doesn't have to be a tedious process. With these simple and practical tips, you can easily incorporate nutritious and delicious meals into your busy lifestyle. Remember to choose versatile recipes, batch cook/prep ingredients, invest in the right kitchen tools, and think of meal prep as a way to strengthen the foundation for a healthier life. Don't strive for perfection, but instead focus on consistent and incremental improvements.

CHAPTER 8

Meal Timing and Frequency for Optimal Results

"The timing of your meals is just as important as what you're eating."

Meal timing isn't just another health fad. Think of it as powerful as managing your finances—it's all about making strategic choices. Eating at the right times can boost your energy, improve your workouts, and balance your blood sugar levels. It simply makes sense.

Ever wonder why some people seem to bounce back so quickly after a workout? It's all in the timing. Eating a balanced meal or snack before and after your workout can work wonders. Before exercising, **carbohydrates** give you the energy to power through.

Protein, on the other hand, is the building block your muscles need after you've given them a good workout. A simple yet effective combo - **a banana and a handful of nuts before hitting the gym**, and perhaps **a protein shake afterwards**.

Skipping meals might seem like a quick fix, but it's more like pulling the battery out of a clock and expecting it to keep time. Spacing your meals evenly throughout the day keeps you ticking smoothly. Regular meals help maintain **stable blood sugar levels**, preventing those mid-afternoon energy crashes that leave you reaching for junk food.

We all have an internal clock known as the circadian rhythm. It influences everything from our sleep patterns to our metabolism. Eating in sync with your circadian rhythm means having meals at regular intervals and not too late at night. Think of it this way - eating when your body expects food helps it process nutrients more efficiently.

Consider Hugh Jackman, known for his rigorous fitness routines. He often talks about how meal timing played a critical role in his transformation for roles like "Wolverine." Jackman followed a strategy of eating every 2-3 hours, balancing his macronutrients wisely. This approach helps to maintain his lean physique and high energy levels.

By now, you're seeing the patterns. Meal timing isn't about adding complexity to your life; it's about finding rhythm and balance. Understand your body's needs and align them with your activities. This strategy will help you achieve optimal results without the guesswork. It's practical, straightforward, and it works.

Intermittent Fasting

Ever wondered why some people manage to stay in great shape well into their golden years? One key strategy is intermittent fasting (IF). Think of it like giving your body a chance to reset and optimize. Intermittent fasting isn't a diet but a pattern of eating. It tells your body when to eat and when to rest, allowing it to operate at its best.

Your body is designed to adapt. When you fast, your body has time to repair and rejuvenate. Research shows that intermittent fasting can improve metabolism, aid weight loss, and enhance cellular repair.

Your body, during a fasting period, starts to burn fat for energy. This is like flipping a switch from "store mode" to "burn mode." Studies, like the one from the *New England Journal of Medicine*, show that intermittent fasting can help reduce inflammation and boost metabolism.

Intermittent fasting is versatile. Here are a few popular ways -

1. **16/8 Method** - Fast for 16 hours and eat within an 8-hour window. It's simple. Fast overnight and eat from noon to 8 PM.

2. **5 -2 Diet** - Eat normally for five days a week and limit calorie intake (about 500–600 calories) on two non-consecutive days.

3. **Alternate-Day Fasting** - Eat every other day. It's intense but effective for some.

Every method aims for the same result—giving your body a break from constant digestion so it can focus on other vital functions.

Look at Terry Crews, the actor and former NFL player. At age 50, Crews maintains an impressive physique, thanks partly to intermittent fasting. He follows the 16/8 method, only eating from 2 PM to 10 PM. This routine aligns with his busy schedule and intense workouts, helping him maintain his energy levels and muscle mass.

Start with modest adjustments. If you're used to eating breakfast at 7 AM, try pushing it to 9 AM. Gradually extend your fasting period. Listen to your body and ensure you're hydrated. (*Note - Intermittent fasting isn't for everyone. Consult your doctor if you have any medical conditions.*)

Remember, *what* you eat during your eating window is crucial. Fill your meals with nutrient-dense foods - lean proteins, healthy fats, and plenty of vegetables. Avoid empty calories and processed foods. Your body needs quality fuel.

Here's a quick breakdown -

- **Before 2 PM** - Water, black coffee, or tea.
- **2 PM - 10 PM** - Balanced meals. Example - Grilled chicken, quinoa, and a salad with avocado for lunch; salmon and roasted vegetables for dinner.

Intermittent fasting is a tool, not a cure-all. The goal is to create a sustainable routine that fits your lifestyle. It should enhance your life, not complicate it. Keep track of how you feel. Adjust as necessary.

Taking Control of Your Nutrition – Timing is Everything

Understanding nutrient timing can change the way you approach fitness after 50. It's like having an internal clock that knows exactly when to eat to boost your performance and recovery. The key is to fuel your body when it needs it most—before and after a workout. Let's break this down into what everyone should know.

Take LeBron James, for instance. At age 39, he's still dominating the basketball court. One of his secrets? Strategic nutrient timing. He makes sure to fuel up before games and recover right after. This routine keeps him in peak condition, both on and off the court.

You don't have to be an athlete to benefit from these principles. Plan your meals around your workouts. Start small. Adjust as you learn what works best for you. Keep it practical.

Example meal plan -

- **Morning Workout** - Have a smoothie with Greek yogurt and berries an hour before.
- **After Workout** - Eat a turkey sandwich on whole-grain bread.

Nutrient timing isn't just a trend; it's backed by science. Dr. John Ivy, a prominent exercise physiologist, has done extensive research on this topic. His studies show that nutrient timing can improve your body's response to exercise and enhance muscle recovery.

Listen to your body. Everyone's different. You may need to tweak the timing a bit to find what works best for you. The goal is to make these practices part of your routine. Small, consistent changes will yield significant results over time.

Addressing Common Concerns and Misconceptions About Meal Timing

When it comes to meal timing, there's a lot of noise out there. It's easy to get lost in myths and misinformation. Let's cut through the clutter.

Myth - Eating More Frequently Boosts Metabolism

This is a popular one, but it's not as straightforward as it seems. Consuming multiple small meals throughout the day won't necessarily fire up your metabolism. What truly matters is your overall calorie intake and the quality of your food. For example, a study from the University of Ottawa showed that people who ate three balanced meals a day had no difference in metabolic rate compared to those who ate six smaller meals. *Quality over quantity.*

Myth - Skipping Breakfast Wrecks Your Metabolism

Many believe that skipping breakfast is a surefire way to pack on the pounds. While having a wholesome breakfast can kickstart your day, missing it won't doom your metabolism. However, the risk lies in potentially overeating later. Think of breakfast as setting the tone for the day, but it's your total daily intake that counts. Listen to your body's signals. If you aren't hungry, it's okay to skip.

Myth - Fasting Leads to Nutrient Deficiencies

There's worry about missing out on essential nutrients when fasting. If planned well, intermittent fasting can be incredibly beneficial. With a shorter eating window, you become more conscious of what you eat. You're more likely to prioritize whole, nutrient-dense foods to meet your body's needs. Focus on quality and variety within your meals.

Myth - Late-Night Eating Equals Weight Gain

We've all heard, "Don't eat after 8 PM." The truth? Timing isn't as crucial as total energy balance. Imagine trying to fill a bucket. It doesn't matter when you pour; what matters is how much. Studies, like one from Northwestern University, have shown that what and how much you eat is more important than when you eat it. If you're hungry at night, opt for something like a small yogurt or a piece of fruit. Keep it light and nutritious.

Myth - Fasting Affects Exercise Performance

Some fear they won't perform well exercising on an empty stomach. While fasted workouts can be challenging, they also offer benefits. For instance, endurance athletes often train fasted to enhance fat burning.

On the flip side, it's also essential to refuel post-exercise. Again, consider basketball legend LeBron James, who follows a balanced diet to maintain peak performance. If you're fasting, aim to eat a meal rich in protein and carbs after your workout to aid recovery.

There's no one-size-fits-all. Your lifestyle, preferences, and goals should dictate your approach. Stay informed, listen to your body, and choose what works best for you.

It's never too late to take control of your health. With clarity comes action. And with action, progress. In conclusion, meal timing and frequency are like finding the right tempo in music. Consistency, quality, and listening to your body's signals are key to harmonizing your eating habits with your goals.

CHAPTER 9

Hydration and Its Impact on Lean Muscle Maintenance

"Hydration is the driving force of all nature."
Leonardo da Vinci

Water is not just a thirst quencher. It's the lifeline of your muscle cells. **At least 60% of an adult human body is water**, and muscles hold a large portion of it. **When dehydrated, muscle cells lose volume**, which leads to weakness and fatigue. Proper hydration ensures muscles work efficiently, helps in protein synthesis, and even aids in muscle recovery after workouts.

Let's talk numbers. Even a **1-2% loss in body water** can cause significant drops in physical performance. One study featured by the *Journal of Athletic Training* highlighted that dehydrated athletes showed a decrease in strength, power, and high-intensity endurance by 20%. This drop can make everyday activities and workouts much harder for you.

So, how much water do you need? That's a **loaded question**. In this chapter, we'll dive into the science of hydration and its impact on lean muscle maintenance. From understanding your individual needs to replenishing electrolytes post-workout, you'll learn how to keep yourself properly hydrated for optimal health and fitness.

Sippin' Smart - Water for Muscles!

We've all heard it - drink more water. But have you ever wondered just how deeply hydration impacts your journey towards staying fit and maintaining muscle, especially as we age? Let's explore this real quick, with a few examples to make it relatable.

Water is your body's natural fuel. It helps number 1, digest food, number 2, regulate temperature, and number 3, moves nutrients to where they need to go. When you're hydrated, everything works better. Without enough water, you might find yourself confused, and slow, and that's not just in your workouts, but in daily life too.

When you workout, you sweat. And with sweat, your body loses not just water, but essential electrolytes. This can throw off your whole system. Dehydration reduces blood volume which makes your heart work harder. Studies show that dehydrated muscles fatigue quicker. Imagine running on empty; that's your muscles without water.

Muscles are like sponges, and they need water to stay flexible and strong. Think of hydration as the foundation for muscle recovery and growth. Water helps deliver nutrients to muscles and removes waste. Without enough of it, muscles can cramp, and you'll feel more sore after workouts. That's why staying hydrated can actually make your workouts less painful and more productive.

Believe it or not, dehydration affects your brain too. Picture trying to think through a fog. Mild dehydration can impair short-term memory, attention, and mental function. Adequate water intake helps keep your mind sharp and focused, which is especially important when you're tackling new fitness challenges.

Heavy exercise or hot weather poses a real risk for dehydration. Let's not go into a tailspin thinking about it, but yes, there's a chance of heat-related illnesses. Staying hydrated helps you avoid these risks by keeping your body at the right temperature.

If there's one quick tip to share, it's this - keep a water bottle with you always. Don't wait until you're thirsty because that's your body already calling for help.

Sip Up, Shape Up

Let's dive into a scenario we all can relate to. Imagine running a marathon when you haven't trained for a day. Tough, right? Now, consider your body in this scenario when it's not properly hydrated. It's a similar struggle.

First things first, staying hydrated is more than just drinking water when you're thirsty. *Thirst is a late indicator of dehydration.* Aim for around *8 glasses of water a day.* You've probably heard this before, but it's true!

Picture yourself gardening for hours under the summer sun. Your body is like a garden that needs watering.

Dehydration can leave you feeling fatigued even with light physical activities.

1. **Drink Water Regularly** - Don't wait until you're parched. Make it a habit to drink water frequently throughout the day. **Carry a reusable water bottle** everywhere you go. Little sips go a long way.

2. **Watch Your Urine Color** - Here's an easy trick. If your urine is pale yellow or straw-colored, you're good. Darker urine? Time to drink more water. It's a simple, effective self-check.

3. **Hydrate Around Workouts** - Drink a glass of water *before* you start exercising. Take small sips during your workout. After you're done, rehydrate to help with recovery. Years ago, the Gatorade Sports Science Institute studied athletes. They found that those who were well-hydrated had reduced muscle soreness and better performance. This isn't just for top athletes; it applies to all of us.

4. **Consider Electrolytes** - If you're engaged in prolonged or high-intensity activities, you might need to replace electrolytes too. Sodium and potassium are key here. Sports drinks or supplements can help.

5. **Hydrating Foods** - Watermelon, cucumbers, strawberries, and oranges. These are not just delicious; they're high in water content and a great addition to your diet. An easy win for hydration.

6. **Mind the Booze and Caffeine** - Too much alcohol and caffeine can dehydrate you. If you indulge, balance it with extra water.

7. **Adjust for Weather** - Hot days demand more fluids. Sweat more, drink more. Simple math.

You're fueling your entire body. It keeps your mind sharp too. Dehydration can mess with your cognition, making it harder to stay focused and make decisions.

Different Fluids for Hydration

You know, it's easy to think hydration is just about guzzling down water. But let's dive into some drinks that might surprise you and clear up a few common myths.

You just finished a morning walk. It's hot, you're sweating, and reaching for a drink. Here's the lowdown on what to pick -

1. **Water** - The obvious choice. Zero calories. Instantly hydrating. Always keep a bottle handy. Aim for about *eight glasses a day.*

2. **Sports Drinks** - Useful if you're sweating buckets from a long session. They replace electrolytes you lost. Key here is moderation; most store-bought ones can have extra sugars you don't need unless you're running marathons like Eliud Kipchoge. If he uses them for records, you can use them for tough gym sessions.

3. **Coconut Water** - Think of it as nature's sports drink. Packed with potassium and low in sugar compared to sports drinks. Imagine you've had a rigorous Pilates class; this can help replenish lost minerals.

4. **Herbal Teas** - Ginger tea for cold days or iced peppermint tea in summer. No calories, full of flavor. And ginger tea can soothe inflammation.

5. **Milk** - Underappreciated! Post-exercise, it's a fantastic recovery drink. You get hydration plus calcium and protein, essential for bone and muscle strength.

Busting Hydration Myths

Imagine you're starting your day with a brisk morning walk. It's sunny and warm, and by the end, you're sweating. You head home, grab a glass of water, and feel accomplished. But there's more to hydration than just drinking water, and it's crucial for maintaining lean muscle after 50.

Let's debunk some common myths that could be holding you back.

Myth 1 - Only Water Hydrates

It's a hot day, and you're tempted by a sports drink. You might think, "But isn't water the only real way to hydrate?" Actually, other beverages can hydrate just as well. Milk, for instance, not only hydrates but also provides protein, calcium, and essential nutrients vital for muscle maintenance. A study from McMaster University found that milk could be more effective than some sports drinks for post-exercise recovery, particularly in promoting muscle growth.

Myth 2 - Older Adults Need Less Water

Many believe that as we age, we need less water. This is false. Our bodies still need consistent hydration. The issue is that thirst signals weaken with age, making it easy to overlook dehydration. Even mild dehydration can impair cognitive function and physical performance. Older adults need to be proactive about their fluid intake, sipping water regularly throughout the day.

Myth 3 - Coffee Dehydrates You

Everyone loves a good cup of coffee. But isn't it dehydrating? Surprisingly, moderate coffee consumption contributes to your fluid intake. According to a study by the University of Birmingham, the diuretic effect of caffeine is mild and doesn't negate the hydration benefits. So, enjoy your morning coffee knowing it's helping, not hindering, your hydration goals.

Myth 4 - Hydration Only Matters in Hot Weather

Hydration is essential year-round, not just in the summer. Dehydration can occur in any climate, impacting health and performance. Think of it like oil for your car engine;

without proper hydration, your body can't function smoothly. Winter months can be particularly deceptive, as the lack of heat reduces our thirst prompting. Always keep a water bottle handy, whether it's January or July.

When you can't live without it, you might as well make it work for you. Hydration is vital to overall health and well-being, and now you know the real deal about different beverages and hydration myths.

CHAPTER 10

Overcoming Plateaus and Adapting to Change

"It is not the strongest of the species that survives, nor the most intelligent, but the one most responsive to change."
Charles Darwin

We've all been there. You're putting in the effort, hitting the gym regularly, eating right, but progress just seems to stall. It's like running into a wall. But here's the truth - plateaus *are* part of the process. They challenge us to adapt and push beyond our limits.

Think about Tom Hanks. Yes, the Hollywood actor. Before he played Captain Miller in "Saving Private Ryan", Tom had to undergo intense physical training. Despite his age, he was 41 back then, he faced the brutal boot camps and conditioning. There were days when he felt beaten, but he adapted his training, persisted, and gave a stellar performance.

You might not be prepping for a war film, but the principles apply. Recognize that a plateau is not a failure. It's feedback. Your body has adapted to your current routine, and it's time to mix it up. Shift your workout regimen, try different exercises, increase the intensity, or perhaps change your diet. The keys here are adaptability and persistence.

There's a powerful concept in psychology known as the "Growth Mindset", coined by Carol Dweck. Those with a growth mindset see challenges as opportunities. They believe abilities can be developed through dedication and hard work. **This mindset is crucial when overcoming plateaus.**

To sum it all up, plateaus are detours, not dead ends. In this chapter, we'll explore strategies to overcome plateaus and adapt to change. Because growth happens when we step out of our comfort zone.

Shattering Fitness and Nutrition Plateaus

One common misconception is that plateaus mean you've done something wrong. That's not true. They simply mean your body has adapted. This is a good thing. It shows progress. Now, it's time to change things up. By tweaking your routines, you can jumpstart your progress again.

Imagine your body as a machine, one that's gotten very good at conserving energy. When you keep doing the same exercises, it finds ways to do them more efficiently, using fewer resources. That's why variety is key.

Instead of always walking, try adding weight training or yoga. Mixing up your exercises can trick your body out of its comfort zone. Studies by the American Council on Exercise show that varying workouts helps in maintaining muscle growth and overall fitness.

If you've been lifting the same weights or running the same distance, it's time to up the ante. Push a little harder. Increase weights by 10% or add a few more minutes to your cardio session each week. High-intensity interval training (HIIT) can be particularly effective.

Nutrition - Small Tweaks, Big Impact

Diet isn't just about what you eat, but also how and when you eat. Small adjustments can lead to significant results.

As we age, our metabolism changes. Keep an eye on your protein, fats, and carbs. Protein, especially, is crucial for muscle repair and growth. Dr. John Ivy, a renowned sports nutritionist, suggests that older adults need more protein to maintain their muscle mass—around 1.2 grams per kilogram of body weight daily.

Breaking through plateaus often starts in your head. If you believe a plateau is a dead end, it becomes one. But if you see it as a sign of progress, you'll approach it differently.

Consistency over Perfection - Being steady with your efforts is more important than doing things perfectly. Remember, progress isn't linear. Celebrate small wins and keep going.

In summary, plateaus aren't your enemy. They are signposts, guiding you to adapt and innovate. Change your workouts, tweak your diet, and shift your mindset. You'll not only break through those barriers but will also come out stronger on the other side.

Resilience in the Face of Setbacks

There will be highs and lows. Famous cases like that of Ernestine Shepherd, the world's oldest competitive female bodybuilder, illustrate that perseverance pays off. She didn't start bodybuilding until she was 56. By 74, she was a world record holder. It's about seeing setbacks as part of the path.

View setbacks not as failures, but as valuable lessons. In 2013, Bill Gates said it's fine to celebrate success, but it's more important to heed the lessons of failure. Apply this mindset to fitness - each setback teaches you something about your body's limits and potentials.

Even small victories deserve celebration. Did you manage to lift a heavier weight this week? That's progress. Tracking small milestones keeps you motivated. A study from Harvard Business School found that recognizing small achievements boosts overall motivation significantly.

Gratitude turns what we have into enough. Acknowledge your body for what it can do. A study published in the Journal of Personality and Social Psychology states that gratitude can improve mental and emotional well-being. Take a moment every day to thank your body for its strength and resilience.

Visualize your success. Michael Phelps, the most decorated Olympian of all time, used visualization as a critical part of his training. Seeing yourself overcoming challenges sets a positive tone and keeps you focused. Dream big, but take realistic steps.

Resilience in fitness isn't about avoiding failures; it's about learning, adapting, and moving forward. Through these strategies, you can face any setback, stay motivated, and achieve long-term success, just like Ernestine did.

CHAPTER 11

Rest and Recovery for Optimal Health and Performance

"Rest and recovery are not the same as idleness."
Alex Soojung-Kim Pang

You're training hard, lifting weights, hitting the pavement for those morning runs. But something's missing. You're feeling sluggish, even though you're pushing yourself. Your body is like a high-performance machine. It needs time to cool down, to recharge. Without proper rest, you risk burning out.

Remember, rest and recovery aren't weaknesses. In this final chapter, we'll explore the importance of rest and recovery in maintaining optimal health and performance.

Cracking the Code to Recharge: Sleep, Stress, and Recovery Essentials

Imagine pushing a well-oiled machine to its limits without ever shutting it down for maintenance. Eventually, it falters. Similarly, our bodies aren't designed to operate non-stop. Especially as we age, rest and recovery become indispensable components of a fitness journey.

Dr. Matthew Walker, a leading expert on sleep, found that even partial sleep deprivation can impact cognitive functions and increase inflammation. Imagine trying to train not only physically tired but mentally foggy, too. His research shows those who sleep well have healthier hearts and sharper minds. Simple changes can make a difference. Try keeping a consistent sleep schedule and limit screen time before bed.

Your body communicates its needs. Feelings of fatigue, soreness, and lethargy are signs that you need rest. Overtraining can lead to burnout, making it crucial to tune in. Trust your body's signals. If you need a break, take it.

Imagine LeBron James skipping sleep before a game—unthinkable, right? Sleep is that essential. Aim for 7 to 9 hours each night. During deep sleep, your body repairs tissues, grows muscles, and synthesizes vital hormones.

Life throws curveballs, but chronic stress shouldn't derail your fitness journey. High cortisol levels from prolonged stress can lead to weight gain. Stress isn't just about feeling overwhelmed. It's a chemical reaction. Dr. Jon Kabat-Zinn's research on mindfulness shows that just *10 minutes* of daily meditation can lower stress hormones. Find what relaxes you. Maybe it's yoga, journaling, or simply a walk in nature. Set aside some "me time" daily.

Contrary to popular belief, recovery isn't just sitting still. Active recovery is your friend. Low-intensity exercises like walking, swimming, or yoga keep the blood flowing and speed up recovery. A yoga practice as short as *20 minutes* can significantly improve flexibility, according to Harvard Health.

Jane, a 55-year-old runner and client of mine, incorporated yoga into her regimen and noticed fewer injuries. Her flexibility improved, and so did her race times. This isn't coincidence; it's science-backed practice.

Your body communicates its needs clearly—fatigue, soreness, and lethargy are all signals. Overtraining leads to burnout. A rest day is not laziness; it's wisdom. Former Olympian Carl Lewis credits part of his success to listening to his body and not overtraining.

When you feel signs of overreaching, ease off. Maybe it's time for a lighter workout or complete rest. Trust these signals. They are your guide to sustained fitness.

Mastering Relaxation and Mindfulness

When it comes to relaxation, **guided imagery** and **autogenic training** are game-changers. You're sitting in a quiet room, eyes closed, visualizing a serene beach. The sound of the waves calms you. That's guided imagery. It helps manage pain and stress.

Autogenic training is a bit different. It involves repeating phrases to yourself, like "My arms are heavy," which can trigger a calming response in your body. These practices reduce stress and improve sleep quality, enhancing your recovery process.

Mindfulness isn't just for monks. It's practical and powerful. Seated meditation, especially for those with limited mobility, is an excellent start. Sit comfortably, close your eyes, and focus on your breathing. Just 10 minutes a day can decrease anxiety and improve focus. Take Carl Lewis, for example. The legendary track and field athlete credits part of his success to mindfulness. His routines helped him stay centered and perform consistently.

Digital detox is crucial. Set aside specific times to turn off your gadgets. This reduces stress from constant connectivity, helping you sleep better.

Activities like knitting or painting aren't just hobbies— they're meditative practices. They help you focus and reduce stress. Then there's music therapy. Listening to calm music or nature sounds can reduce stress hormones and improve brain health. Just look at pianist and composer Ludovico Einaudi. He talks about how playing piano has been his meditation and therapy, helping him manage stress and stay creative.

Creating an Optimal Sleep Environment

Creating a sleep haven isn't just some fluffy talk; it's backed by science. For those of us in our golden years, getting good rest is like hitting the reset button on our bodies and minds. Let's break it down.

You're in your late 50s, and you've just discovered the magic of *blackout curtains*. It's more than just a decor choice. By blocking out all unwanted light, these curtains signal to your brain that it's time to shut down and sleep deeply. Scientific studies have shown that darkness triggers the production of melatonin, a hormone that regulates sleep. You fall asleep faster and enjoy a more restful night.

Now, let's talk temperature. You're not 25 anymore, and your body's thermostat needs a little extra help. A cool room, ideally between 60-67 degrees Fahrenheit, can significantly improve your sleep quality. Think of it as your personal 'sleep cave.' Lowering the room temperature helps your body signal that it's time to rest, much like it does naturally as the sun goes down.

As we age, our needs change. Investing in a mattress and pillows that cater to your body's specific support requirements can be a game-changer. *Research suggests* that a good mattress can reduce back and neck pain, common culprits for waking up at night. Don't skimp on this—it's an investment in your health. Replace your mattress every 7-10 years and choose pillows that provide solid neck support.

Noise can be a sleep killer. If you live in a noisy area, consider earplugs or a white noise machine. These tools mask disruptive sounds and create a consistent auditory environment, lulling you into deeper sleep. Imagine living next to a bustling street. A white noise machine can cancel out the honking and chatter, replacing it with soothing, consistent sounds that your brain can tune out.

Let's not forget tech. It's tempting to scroll through your phone before bed, but this habit might be your worst enemy. The blue light emitted by screens messes with your melatonin levels. Oprah Winfrey, a huge advocate for mental well-being, often emphasizes the importance of a tech break before sleep. Set a 'digital sunset'—turn off your gadgets at least an hour before you plan to hit the sack.

In summary, aligning your sleep environment with these principles can bring substantial improvement to your rest quality. Each of these changes might seem small, but together, they create a powerhouse of sleep-enhancing habits. Remember, it's all about building a sanctuary for your sleep. You'll wake up rejuvenated and ready to tackle the day with vigor.

Conquering Sleep Issues

Dealing with sleep disturbances can feel like an uphill battle, but with the right approach, you can reclaim your nights and power through your days. Let's dive into some of the most common sleep disruptors and practical, science-backed strategies to overcome them.

Sleep Apnea

Imagine waking up exhausted despite spending eight hours in bed. That's life with sleep apnea. It's more common than you think, especially as we age. Studies show nearly one in four men and one in ten women over 50 suffer from it. Symptoms include loud snoring, gasping, or daytime fatigue.

If you or your partner notice these signs, consult a healthcare provider. Using a CPAP device might seem daunting, but it can drastically improve your sleep quality and overall health. Think of it like getting a regular night's sleep for the first time in years.

Restless Legs

Restless Legs Syndrome (RLS) feels like an unending itch deep in your legs, urging you to move them constantly. This can make falling asleep a real challenge. RLS affects about 10% of people over 50. The good news? There are ways to manage it.

Cutting back on alcohol and caffeine helps. Moderate exercise, like a 30-minute walk earlier in the day, can ease symptoms too. If these solutions don't work, there are medications that can help. Consult your doctor for options.

Nocturia

Frequent nighttime trips to the bathroom, known as nocturia, can break up your sleep quite literally. Reducing fluid intake a couple of hours before going to bed can help. Also, watch your diet for diuretics like caffeine or alcohol.

Nocturia can sometimes result from underlying conditions like diabetes or bladder issues. An honest conversation with your doctor can rule out these possibilities and lead to effective treatments.

Insomnia

Insomnia often stems from stress, anxiety, or depression, and it becomes more common as we age. You're not alone if you find yourself staring at the ceiling at 2 AM, mind racing. Establishing a relaxing pre-sleep routine can make all the difference. For instance, reading a book or meditating for 15-20 minutes can signal to your brain that it's time to wind down.

Consider Cognitive Behavioral Therapy for Insomnia (CBT-I). It's more effective in the long run than sleep medications, according to a study published in JAMA. It teaches you how to create good sleep habits and challenge the fears that keep you awake.

Building Your Sleep Routine

Let's start with one of the basics - a regular sleep schedule. Consistency is key. Think of your body like a finely-tuned orchestra, responding to a precise conductor—the circadian rhythm. Going to bed and waking up at the same time each day, even on weekends, keeps this internal clock steady. Studies show people sticking to regular hours report better sleep quality and less daytime drowsiness.

Naps can be a double-edged sword. A quick 20-minute nap can refresh your mind and body. Beyond that, and you risk deep sleep, making it harder to nod off at night. If you must nap, do it early afternoon. Remember Ronald Reagan? He loved a brief nap, calling it revitalizing. Follow his lead, but don't overdo it.

Pay attention to what you consume before bed. Large meals can cause discomfort, making it harder to fall asleep. Instead, opt for light snacks, if hungry. And then there's the caffeine factor. A cup of coffee in the afternoon might seem harmless, but it can stay in your system for hours, disrupting sleep. John Hopkins Medicine suggests avoiding caffeine at least six hours before bedtime. Alcohol might make you drowsy, but can lead to fragmented sleep later in the night. Aim to limit fluids in the evening to avoid waking up frequently.

Consider Jeff Bezos. Yes, the Amazon founder. He prioritizes eight hours of sleep a night. Despite his busy schedule, Bezos emphasizes sleep as a critical aspect of his daily routine. He believes it enhances decision-making and creativity. This approach can be mimicked by anyone, proving that prioritizing sleep gives you a leg up in daily performance.

Creating an ideal sleep environment is more tangible than you think. Removing electronic screens an hour before bed helps—blue light can inhibit melatonin production. Make your bedroom a sleep sanctuary - cool, dark, and quiet. Invest in a quality mattress and pillows—your back will thank you. If noise is an issue, earplugs or a white noise machine might offer relief.

Optimizing sleep is not fluff; it's a foundational step to improving health. By instilling these habits, older adults can experience rejuvenated and restorative sleep, leading to better physical health, sharper cognitive abilities, and a mood boost. Imagine waking up each day feeling refreshed, motivated, and ready to conquer whatever comes your way. All it takes is a commitment to a few small changes. Start now, and thrive like Ronald Reagan in his vibrant routines or Jeff Bezos in his creative peak. Your best self awaits.

Conclusion

Turning the Page to a New You

Remember the frustrations that brought you here? Struggling to keep fit as the years went by. Seeing the scale creep up, inch by frustrating inch. Feeling more tired, less energetic. You worried about your health, and maybe even your future. You weren't alone. Many just like you felt the same. You wanted change but didn't know where to start. That's where this journey began.

We dove deep into how to stay lean and healthy after 50. This book tackled the myths and misinformation, shining light on what really works. We discussed the critical importance of maintaining muscle and the role of nutrition. We explored how to adapt exercise routines to your changing body. The goal was always clear: *helping you take back control and achieve your best self.*

Throughout this journey, we knew that change is challenging, but you've shown the willingness to learn and adapt. This wasn't a quick fix or a temporary solution. This was about creating lasting habits. We wanted you to feel empowered, informed, and ready to face the future with confidence.

So, where are you now? Imagine waking up with energy. Imagine feeling strong, capable, and in control of your body. That's what awaits you if you stay on this path. You've gained an understanding of how important it is to keep active and eat right, no matter your age. You've learned to listen to your body, respond to its needs, and push it to new heights. These aren't just physical changes but mental ones too. With every step forward, you've built resilience and a new sense of self-worth.

Understanding that aging isn't an obstacle but an opportunity is liberating. It's a mindset shift. Think of celebrities like Samuel L. Jackson or Helen Mirren, who continually redefine aging gracefully. They've adapted lifestyles that keep them vibrant and active. Take their example to heart. Age is just a number, and your journey has only begun.

Revisiting our thesis, this book was born out of a need to offer real, tangible advice for those over 50. We aimed to dispel myths and provide practical, scientifically-backed information. You now know that staying lean isn't about drastic diets but smart choices. It's about consistency and understanding how your body works.

Let's recall what we covered. **We talked about the vital role of protein** and how it helps maintain muscle mass. You learned the importance of regular strength training and how it fights age-related muscle loss. You discovered the nuances of hydration and its impact on vitality. *We debunked fad diets* and emphasized a balanced, nutrient-dense eating plan. All these takeaways are powerful tools in your arsenal.

Now, it's your turn. Armed with this knowledge, you hold the keys to a healthier future. This is your call to action. Take the principles you've learned and make them part of your life. Start today—your future self will thank you. Imagine being the example others look up to, showing that even after 50, you can be at your best. The journey doesn't end here; it's a continuous evolution. So, keep pushing, keep striving, and most importantly, keep believing in yourself.

Your adventure into fitness and longevity is an inspiring story yet to be fully told. Every choice you make is another chapter. Make it a tale of triumph. Stay lean, stay strong, stay you.

www.ingramcontent.com/pod-product-compliance
Lightning Source LLC
Chambersburg PA
CBHW071038250726
48653CB00005B/1892